CW00683592

"In MAN of IRON, *Kris Gethin displays extreme focus and tenacity in the pursuit of his goals. Kris is a true bodybuilding expert, and he applies his laser-like focus to this IRONMAN endeavor with unmatched precision and intensity. Read Man of IRON for insight into not only a successful IRONMAN training program for hybrid athletes, but also the unique mind of Kris Gethin himself.*"

-ULISSES JR.
2x Musclemania SuperBody Pro Champion,
2x Musclemania World Pro Champion, Celebrity Trainer,
Fitness Entrepreneur, Motivator

"*When Kris approached us letting us know he was about to embark on this Man of Iron project, there were a thousand questions in my head. Ambitious goals mean nothing without execution. The loftiest, greatest goals are noble things to shoot for, but they too easily give us an excuse to quit. Shoot for the moon and even if you'll miss, you'll land amongst the stars, so the saying goes. But that is not the mindset that takes you to the finish. The mindset you'll need is one of dogged, passionate pursuit of the final objective. Attention paid to every single detail, no matter how small. The drive to put in the work precisely on the days you want to quit- when you want to quit, when you tell yourself you can quit and nobody would blame you. The unwillingness to accept anything less than full execution of everything you set out to achieve. From the first training session with him, I knew Kris had all the pieces he'd need to walk across that finish line as a true MAN OF IRON, as the only thing larger than his goals is his own will- his own drive and determination. It was an honor and privilege to be a part of this journey with him, and to see him inspire so many others to set and smash their own personal challenges.*"

-ALEX VIADA CSCS
Founder and head coach, Complete Human Performance,
IRONMAN Competitor, Powerlifter

"During my 30 years on the microphone at IRONMAN events all over the world, I thought I'd seen every imaginable shape and size. But watching Kris enter the water at IRONMAN Coeur d'Alene stopped me short. How could this guy carry that much muscle around for 140.6 miles of swim, bike, and run? But carry it he did, and every mile with a big smile on his face. Calling Kris an IRONMAN at the finish line was a real thrill, and it taught me and everyone watching something important about misconceptions and power of the human spirit."

-MIKE REILLY
"Voice of IRONMAN" and Author of *Finding My Voice: Tales from IRONMAN, the World's Greatest Endurance Event*

"There is literally nothing this man can't do. Kris has an impeccable athletic ability about him because of the way he trains; mentally he is one of the strongest humans I know. Not only does he preach the part, but he acts the part. Understanding what it means to be a true hybrid athlete is something Kris has become an expert on. This book will not only inspire you, but cause you to bring forth your full potential in every aspect of your life."

-ASHLEY HORNER
Fitness celebrity, professional fitness competitor, hybrid-athlete, KAGED MUSCLE athlete and triathlete

MAN OF IRON

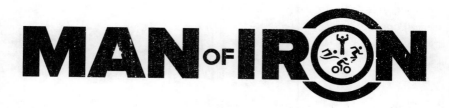

A WORLD CLASS BODYBUILDER'S JOURNEY
TO BECOME AN IRONMAN

Kris Gethin

This book is dedicated to everyone who said bodybuilding, strength training, and powerlifting can't co-exist with triathlon, ultra-marathon, and IRONMAN. This book is evidence that you can. Welcome to Hybrid Athleticism.

INTRODUCTION

As Mike Reilly announced, "Kris Gethin, you are an IRONMAN," goosebumps tingled down my spine. The doubters had finally been silenced. Training for and completing an IRONMAN was one of the most enjoyable challenges I've ever faced, and I'm glad I've proven that with the right program you can build muscle, lose fat, and become an extreme hybrid athlete. In just six months, I was able to attain the physical conditioning required to complete a full IRONMAN in fifteen hours, something which was meant to be "impossible." Further "impossibilities" were overcome as I gained three pounds of lean mass and shed nearly four pounds of fat. That's right—during my IRONMAN training I continued to live as a bodybuilder.

I've written *Man of Iron* to share my journey with you. Throughout this process I became firmly convinced that every endurance athlete should be performing some sort of strength training and every bodybuilder should be performing some sort of cardio/endurance training. Whether you're a former athlete looking to get back into competing and improve your health, a bodybuilder who is curious about incorporating endurance training and a more holistic approach to fitness, or just someone who is interested in learning what it takes to become a MAN of IRON, this book will provide you the necessary tools to become a hybrid athlete and complete an IRONMAN of your own.

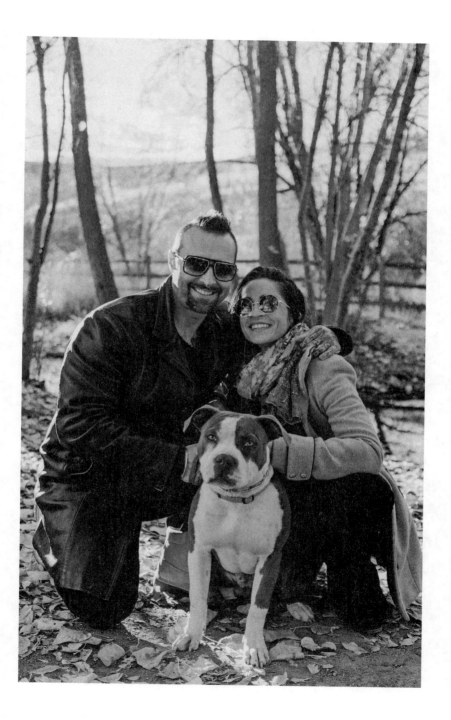

SECTION ONE
SETTING THE STAGE

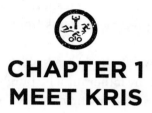

CHAPTER 1
MEET KRIS

My journey to becoming a MAN of IRON started long ago, arguably early in life. My experiences compounded to contribute to my personality, mentality, and life philosophy, each building off each other to lead me to where I am today.

I grew up on a farm in rural Wales, where the sheep outnumber the people. On the farm we had sheep, horses, donkeys, turkeys, and chickens. I didn't have much opportunity to interact with people but didn't miss it, preferring instead to listen to music and read magazines. I started working on the farm from a very young age, which helped to establish structure and a good work ethic. I had to get used to getting up early in the morning—about 6 a.m. I would occasionally work on the farm, have breakfast, and walk a mile up our lane to get the bus to school. It didn't matter if I was walking in knee-deep snow or if it was a beautiful day; I did that every day. Once I got a skateboard, I would walk up as I always did then stash it in the hedgerow so that when I got back from school, I could ride it back down.

My parents were lovingly strict and wanted me to do well, but they didn't put undue pressure on me. I was able to find my strengths based on encouragement from them. If I wanted to make a stupid choice, they would kindly talk me out of it, but they tended to share their perspectives more than barking orders. I was put in my place, and there are times that I probably disliked my father when I was younger, but now I can't thank him enough for being realistic and strict in his discipline. I had (and still have) a lot of respect for my parents, and grew up as a pretty well-behaved kid as a result (they may not agree with this)—and now I definitely wouldn't step out of line as a result of that underlying respect. Much of my discipline in approaching training regimens stems from the early guidance of my parents.

From the time I was about six years old, I became obsessed with motorbikes. I nagged my father until he purchased one for me, and about a year later I entered my first race. Motocross consumed me for approximately the next 15 years. I loved it because it was an individual passion and an individual sport. It was up to me whether I did good or bad, and I had to live with the results. I didn't mind putting pressure on myself; I hated being depended on and depending on others. I work very well alone, and that's why I've always picked up individual-based sports. I've never liked team sports because at the end of the day, you're either a winner or a loser. There's a lot of pressure in team sports, especially in American society, and as a result a lot of people don't participate. They may like the game, they may watch the game, they may go out and practice, but they may never go out and seriously compete because it transitions from being fun and social to being filled with pressure. If you're in an individual sport, such as an IRONMAN or on a bodybuilding stage, if you just finish the event, that can be considered a win. You're competing against yourself and your individual goals.

I absolutely loved motocross. One part of me feared racing because it was nerve-wracking with a lot of pressure, but another part of me was addicted to the adrenaline, to try to excel and improve with every competition. My father probably put me in

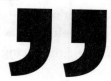

THERE'S A LOT OF PRESSURE IN TEAM SPORTS, ESPECIALLY IN AMERICAN SOCIETY, AND AS A RESULT A LOT OF PEOPLE DON'T PARTICIPATE.

races that were too good for me just so that I could get better faster. I never got comfortable; just as I started to do decent in a certain series of races, we'd go to larger races. Never being at the top developed a chip on my shoulder that has served me well in my quest to explore my athletic potential.

Motocross is one of the most physically demanding sports, which you wouldn't really expect. It works both your anaerobic and aerobic capacities, while utilizing every single muscle in the body at the same time. When you're braking, you're using your triceps, your chest, your shoulders, your stabilizer muscles, your glutes, your hamstrings, your abductors—everything. When you're accelerating, you're using the opposite muscles—your handgrip, your forearms, and your back to stop you from falling backwards. You're always using your abs when you're maneuvering the bike side to side, and you're constantly going over bumps and jumps. It's not as if you're just going up a hill or down a hill—you're maneuvering at the same time. When you're jumping and when you're landing, you tense your legs to hold onto the bike, because a lot of steering is done with your legs. So you're using your core, every primary muscle, every secondary muscle, and every single one of your energy systems for about 40 minutes in a race. When I was young I had a severe case of croup, which weakened my lungs and led me to develop asthma. That asthma always held me back in motocross, to a degree. But I loved the adrenaline from racing, and poured much of my energy into competing.

On top of motocross, I had many different jobs growing up. Obviously, I'd worked on the farm for as long as I could remember, but I started taking up some additional part-time jobs as I grew older. In my teens I worked as a panel beater, an apprentice engineer, a grounds man, a builder's laborer, a wood furniture sander, a driver; I worked in a sawmill, in a furniture warehouse loading trucks; as a barman, a doorman, a lifesaver...I moved from one job to the next quickly. The primary reason for moving between jobs so often was that I felt, personally, that they didn't lead to a place of happiness, motivation, or fulfillment. None of them had good opportunities to move forward. The other reason was that I didn't like the authorities above me, in most instances. I was never really good at being told what to do.

LIFE TAKES A TURN

When I was about 20, I was somewhere within the United Kingdom racing motocross nearly every weekend. It got to the stage where I wasn't able to obtain sponsorship racing motocross, but I could have obtained sponsorship for racing Enduros. Enduros are off-road races lasting as long as several hundred miles over several days, with limited portions being timed. They never did anything for me—they weren't as adrenaline-filled, and they never excited me. At this point, I'd had injuries, namely to my back, so I decided to just hang up the bike and quit racing.

With nothing to work toward, I slipped into a bit of a depression. I started partying, doing drugs, drinking alcohol, and spent time with a social circle that did the same. Motocross is an extreme sport and is surrounded by extreme people, so I just got swept into another extreme culture. As I became depressed, I started putting on weight. I have a major curvature of my spine, which has led to a lot of back problems, and gaining weight put more pressure on my spine, which worsened the pain. It put more pressure on my asthmatic lungs also and, since I was less active, I felt myself starting to spiral out. Drinking and doing drugs created a vicious circle of feeling good under the influence, crashing and coming back to reality, then seeking that high again. I wasn't able to stop, and I could see it was happening with my friends, too.

My back pain reached the point that I started to seek the input of various experts. None could help me until a physical therapist told me I needed to do weight training exercises. These exercises alleviated the stress from my spine through tighter and stronger muscles, and my back actually started to improve—I hadn't realized how bad the pain was until I didn't have it anymore. I felt so much better, and became a significantly happier person as a result. Training became a therapeutic outlet after quitting motocross, and I realized the investment was worth my time. Once I started researching weightlifting and bodybuilding, I found that I was truly interested in learning more, and decided to seek accountability through classes. Remarkably, this was one of the first subjects that I could read all day about and naturally retain.

Growing up I was never any good in school, but a large part of that was due to my lack of interest. I never wanted to learn history. I never wanted to learn about social studies. Not that I've got anything against any type of education—I'd love to absorb it, but I must be sincerely interested if I'm going to retain the information.

Fitness and nutrition genuinely captured my interest and I wasn't easily distracted like I was when reading about most subjects. So, at age 21 I went to college for three years to study international health and sports therapy. In addition, I decided to enter a bodybuilding competition. The combination of my work ethic from the farm and need for that adrenaline fix from motocross was perfect for bodybuilding. I trained my butt off for close to a year and a half. In retrospect, I didn't really know what I was doing. I thought I did—I trained well, I ate very well—but I'd still drink a lot on the weekends because at that point it wasn't something I was able to give up. My friends constantly pressured me. I would initially say no, but inevitably ended out at the pubs with them anyways. However, with eight weeks left until the competition, I put my head down and did everything I could possibly do to succeed and not look like an idiot on that stage.

At that point, I hadn't realized there were tested and untested shows. I didn't know people in the bodybuilding magazines I'd been reading were taking "extracurricular" supplementation or anything

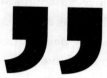

"I DECIDED TO ENTER A BODY-BUILDING COMPETITION. THE COMBINATION OF MY WORK ETHIC FROM THE FARM AND NEED FOR THAT ADRENALINE FIX FROM MOTOCROSS WAS PERFECT FOR BODYBUILDING."

similar. I competed in the show, which was in Pontypridd, Wales, and I was by far the smallest person there. But I'd gotten extremely lean for the show, which really helped my cause, and I was able to place second. I was happy with that, but then I found out most of my competitors were actually on some sort of steroid. I had no idea that's what had to be done to succeed further but after some searching I found drug-tested and polygraph-tested competitions, which I would direct my attention toward for the bodybuilding shows I would later enter in Australia, Canada, and the United States.

At that time I was coming to the end of my college course, and representatives of a company called Steiner came and shared that there were opportunities for people who completed our course to work for their company on cruise liners. I saw a major opportunity—even though I loved Wales and my family, I needed to get away from my social circle and out of the small town that didn't hold opportunities in the direction I wanted to pursue. I joined Steiner and was placed on a five-star celebrity cruise liner for eight months, working as a massage therapist and body therapist. As I came to realize, working on the cruise ship wasn't an escape from the lifestyle I'd tried to leave behind. It was a bigger party than Wales. In the middle of the ocean, with people from different countries, with employee discounts and tax-free purchases, everyone was having a good time and partying virtually every night. It was a lot of fun, but it was very hard work at the same time. I would work 10 to 12 hours a day, with maybe a 30-minute break. Doing that with a hangover wasn't good. But I enjoyed seeing different parts of the world. Employees were commissioned with pay and time off based on how many products they were able to sell. I knew that there were employees on the ship who were better therapists than me, but I was very good at selling, so I got more time off than most. That system didn't sit right with me, and after eight months I decided to pursue a different direction. I'd befriended an Australian while working on the ship, and she invited me to come visit her once I resigned.

MOVING TO THE DOWN UNDER

Within two days of arriving in Sydney, I managed to obtain a job as a floor person at an independent gym called Bodyline, then picked up a couple of part-time jobs on the side as usual. Soon after, I decided to try my hand at starting my own personal training business. For my cardio every day, I would take leaflets advertising my business, which I called Future Physique, and run through neighborhoods posting one into everybody's letterbox. After a couple months I was able to build a decent clientele. I would train people at their homes, or the beach, or the park, and after a while I'd built up a full client base to the extent that my girlfriend, who was also a qualified trainer, had to take on clients as well. I loved waking up and going to train people on the beach at 5 a.m., or in front of the Sydney Opera House. It was a wonderful period in my life.

Around the time my business started to take off, I went to watch a couple bodybuilding shows. At a drug-tested natural bodybuilding show, I saw a man named Mark Kostanti and was blown away. His body showed what can happen to a physique if it's taken care of correctly and fueled with natural food and natural supplementation, and just bloody hard work. I have to admit; in the beginning, I thought there was no way he could be natural. But we became friends, then training partners, and I realized he was just on a different level. My impression of impossibility within the natural sphere turned into possibility after witnessing what Mark could do, and I decided to start competing again, this time within the natural federation. As it turns out, I did quite well, getting second in several shows and qualifying for the Natural World Championships in Toronto, Canada, within four years of my first-ever competition.

With the money that I saved up I purchased a gym in Sydney, which focused purely on either 12-week or 18-week transformations. I didn't want someone to come in, take five personal training sessions, and go—I wanted to see results. I knew that before-and-after pictures from the transformations would help me sell other programs I was developing. My plan worked, and I ran the gym for the next three years while I was competing.

At that time, I realized I wanted to reach more people than just through the one-on-one sessions I offered at the gym. I decided to teach myself writing skills so I could contribute to magazines. I bought Merriam Webster's *Manual for Writers and Editors* and taught myself to write—to a certain degree, at least—and started submitting articles to a number of publications. I also taught myself photography so that I would have photos to accompany the articles, which made it more likely for them to be accepted. Eventually my pieces started to gain traction, and I expanded my scope.

I sold my gym and moved to Venice, California, where I had the opportunity to work for *FLEX Magazine* as a writer and a photographer. After a couple of years, I became a little frustrated at the amount of editing my articles received, and decided to start my own magazine, *Kaged Muscle*. *Kaged Muscle* is what brought me to Boise, Idaho, because the then-CEO of BodyBuilding.com, Ryan Deluca, saw the magazine and offered me the position of editor-in-chief for their website. In 2007 I moved to Boise, and completed my last two years of professional bodybuilding in 2008 and 2009. I placed second in the World Championships, then decided to compete in the Idaho State Titles. I won that show, and realized that I gained no more satisfaction winning than coming in second. I decided to give up bodybuilding as a competitive sport, but I still love to train. Training is very therapeutic for me and always will be.

At Bodybuilding.com, I was still training, and there weren't many employees with the company who were bodybuilding. So Ryan Deluca sort of forced me in front of the camera and said, "You know what you're talking about—you can host our video series." At first I was very uncomfortable and nervous, but over the years I got used to being in front of the camera rather than simply

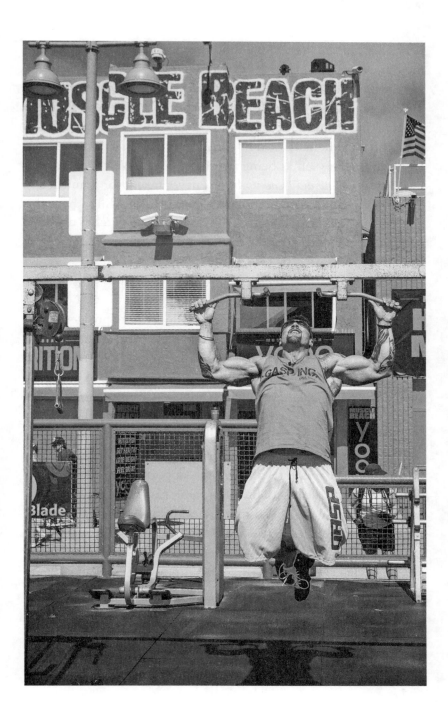

being behind the scenes in editorial, and that transition changed my direction. I can't thank Ryan enough for challenging me and forcing me into the spotlight, because that's given me a higher level of accountability and a higher sense of purpose. It's easier for me to resist taking a day off because there is an expectation from others for me to help them. I love doing that every day. It's strange because I still think of myself as being that farm boy in Wales. Sometimes I ask myself, *How did I end up here?* I never take it for granted, and I'm going to continue doing this as long as I can while I have this platform to help people. Even if only one person watches or shows up, that's great. I'm extremely thankful.

LIFE TAKES ANOTHER TURN

In 2010 I had to return to the United Kingdom due to problems with my visa. It turned out that my lawyer had messed up the paperwork, and despite my best efforts, I was not allowed to live in the United States for several years as I went through the process of obtaining a green card. I was planning to move to Spain in the meantime, but I received a call from my business partner Jag Chima, who told me that a celebrity named Hrithik Roshan was interested in working with me. I'd never heard of this gentleman, but he was a big deal over in India. I was intrigued by the opportunity, and figured I would go over to meet with him. His passion and dedication greatly impressed me, so I decided to work with him. I moved to India, which ended up changing my course in several ways.

I experienced the Indian culture, and enjoyed how different it was from what I was used to. I operate as a very punctual person, and many people in India didn't like to work with me because I wasn't willing to tolerate someone being more than 15 minutes late to an appointment. But I struck up very good relationships with several Bollywood actors based on my success with Hrithik Roshan, which generated more demand. Jag and I started flying in more trainers

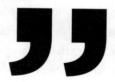

SOMETIMES I ASK MYSELF,
HOW DID I END UP HERE?
I NEVER TAKE IT FOR
GRANTED, AND I'M GOING
TO CONTINUE DOING THIS
AS LONG AS I CAN WHILE
I HAVE THIS PLATFORM
TO HELP PEOPLE.

to work with clients and meet their needs, which led to Jag, myself, and another friend, Neil Hill, developing a certification program in order to educate native Indian trainers and eventually create a franchise of Kris Gethin gyms. Many Indians aren't confident that they can build muscle or fitness because they don't think they have the resources to, nutritional or otherwise. I sought to prove to them that they could, so I created a Muscle Building video series for Bodybuilding.com in which I ate Indian food, trained in Indian gyms, and transformed just the same. Many of the gyms in India did have inferior gym equipment and didn't provide decent education to their trainers, which prompted Jag and I to create a franchise called Kris Gethin Gyms. The Kris Gethin gyms aren't just gyms they're training academies to improve the infrastructure of personal health and fitness in the country. This snowball effect successfully transforms thousands of Indian clientele.

Around the time that I developed my gyms, I saw a need in the marketplace for natural, effective supplements. I'd been creating my own supplements by purchasing various raw materials, and based on the research regarding efficacious dosaging of each ingredient, I would mix my own to achieve the optimal results. This wasn't an ideal process, because mixing and creating these supplements took a lot of time, money, and energy. If I wanted to go out and purchased supplements already on the shelves, they contained artificial flavorings, artificial coloring, dyes, under-dosed ingredients, and generic rather than patented ingredients—and the glutamine and BCAAs were created from either bird feathers or human hair! I didn't want to be putting those things in my body.

I wanted to eat a certain way, train a certain way, and supplement a certain way to benefit my health rather than distracting or taking away from it. Based on hours upon hours of calls, meetings, and conversations with Brian Rand, who I believe is the best formulator in the world, I started traveling to organic farms in places like India and Thailand to see how I might go about sourcing the organic

" I WANTED TO EAT A
CERTAIN WAY, TRAIN
A CERTAIN WAY, AND
SUPPLEMENT A
CERTAIN WAY TO
BENEFIT MY HEALTH
RATHER THAN
DISTRACTING OR
TAKING AWAY FROM IT.

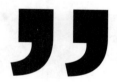

ingredients needed for a natural supplement line. My time spent in the bodybuilding industry had created all the contacts I needed to form the best possible team—I just needed to introduce the right people to each other. I'm fully confident that the business we created, KAGED MUSCLE, has the best team in the world. We started remotely while I was in India and continued when I moved back to Wales as soon as I was granted my American green card. In Wales, I continued to oversee my Indian training programs remotely while filming another trainer video series. KAGED MUSCLE started to gain momentum because all of our products are banned substance certified free, naturally flavored and colored, patented, effectively dosed, and pass Proposition 65 heavy metal contaminant tests, which together comprise more than 600 tests.[1] Many companies aren't willing to put the money into that and focus on marketing instead, but when our products passed all of those tests and proved effective as supplements, people started to pay attention.

With KAGED MUSCLE taking off, I decided it was time to move back to Boise. I could be within striking distance of the KAGED MUSCLE headquarters, I was back in town with Bodybuilding. com, and I got to live the lifestyle I loved in a setting with beautiful nature and great people. Though I didn't realize it at the time, I was perfectly poised to begin the journey toward becoming a hybrid athlete.

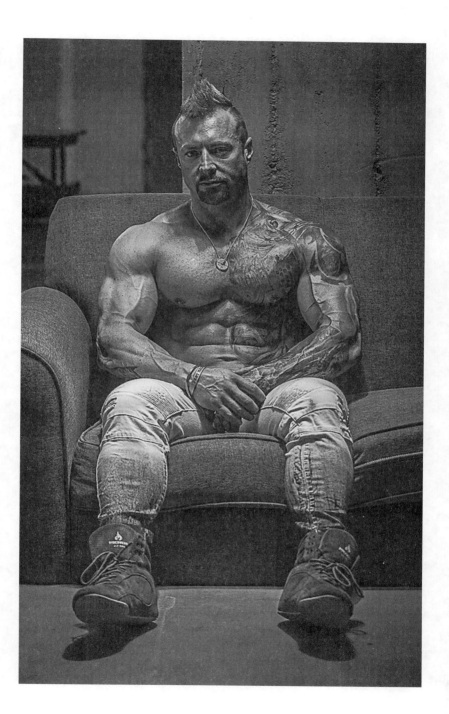

CHAPTER 2
THE IRONMAN DECISION AND FINDING A COACH

The transition to training for this IRONMAN came in different phases and forms. As a bodybuilder, it's easy to get tunnel vision and get stuck in a rut, but I've never found myself in that position. I've always liked to participate in a variety of sports—mountain biking, downhill mountain biking, motocross, surfing, and snowboarding—but I never competed in any of them after starting to body build. Bodybuilding is my passion, and I will never give that up. It helps significantly with the alleviation of my back pain; I develop better bone density, a stronger heart; I lower the risk of heart disease; I improve my energy, confidence, immune system, the list goes on. I do it for therapy and out of necessity. So this IRONMAN was just another sidestep, another challenge for me to pursue.

I became intrigued by triathlons and IRONMANs after I watched some of my friends get into them. A guy I grew up with, Eifion Rees, decided to start doing endurance competitions around 10 years ago. I thought he was crazy. He was losing a lot of his size, which was completely unappealing to me, but at the same time I was very interested in what he was doing because I thought, *He's going to swim how many miles in the water?* I couldn't even swim a length. Then I would see him on an early Sunday afternoon after he had already biked 100 miles in the morning! What he was doing sounded insane, but I was inspired by his dedication. I never thought I could do it because I didn't want to become so small after spending so much time trying to get big and muscular.

Another friend of mine from Wales named Matthew Pritchard puts himself through these crazy intense feats of mental strength and endurance. He would decide to do 30 Half-IRONMANs in 30 days, or he would do three full IRONMANs in three days. And he would do it all for charity and capture it by video and editorial along the way. I was intrigued that someone could put himself or herself into that mental and physical state, not because someone was holding a gun to their head, but because they actually wanted to do it. He was previously a star on a huge MTV show called *Dirty Sanchez*, which was a much more hardcore version of the U.S. version, *Jackass*, so this may have justified his talent for tolerating pain. I couldn't fathom why somebody would want to train so hard for 20-plus hours per week, for many years, just to prepare, but I was inspired by the shock factor—and then I realized it wasn't all that different than what bodybuilders do to their bodies in a gym. It's just a different wiring! Bodybuilders push their bodies to the limit in a short and intense fashion, and endurance guys draw it out—they probably can't do what we do, but we can't do what they do, either.

I reached my tipping point when I read a book called *Iron War*. It chronicles the 1989 IRONMAN World Championship battle between two rivals, Dave Scott and Mark Allen, and it absolutely blew my mind. Mark Allen had barely lost to Dave Scott six years in a row, for various reasons. He was very calculated and technical in everything he did, while Dave Scott was very different. He had less technique and very little natural talent, but he outworked and ou muscled everybody. He was just an animal. A lot of people would comment that he didn't even have the technical correctness to run, but his mental strength would always win. Mark Allen would mostly beat Dave Scott throughout the year at smaller events, but then Dave Scott, a.k.a. "The MAN," would always turn it on when he wanted to with a win at Hawaii, at the world championships, every year. It was in 1989 that they raced neck-and-neck the entire race, both absolutely demolishing their previous personal bests and the rest of the field with it. Mark Allen finally beat Dave Scott for the first time. The story made a huge impact on me. I thought, *Wow. That takes some serious strength and courage. How does someone get beaten all those years and still come back?* These guys were just unbelievable. They had no power meters, no clip-in bike shoes, no special lightweight running shoes as they do today, and a lot of competitors didn't even wear helmets—but only in recent years have their times been beaten. They still have record times within the top 10 of all time today.

POWERING PERFORMANCE WITH MUSCLE

After looking at pictures of most triathletes, I couldn't help but notice how thin they were, and I figured that was what made them so good. I would definitely be awful at something like an IRONMAN, because I outweighed these guys with muscle by 50 or 60 pounds. But a recent study, published in *Medicine and Science in Sports and Exercise,* evaluated the results of maximal strength training for a group of high-level distance runners who were completing their regular endurance training in the same time frame. Researchers found that over eight weeks, the strength training group showed significant improvements in one repetition max testing (33.2%), rate of force development (26%), running economy (5%), and maximal aerobic speed (21.3%), compared to no changes in the control group.[2]

Even though being slender means less weight to carry, the results do show that building muscle can be helpful for triathletes. Regardless, I thought I was too big to be successful at an IRONMAN—so that's when I decided to do it. If I know I'm going to be bad at something, it gives me a big, exciting space of opportunity to improve. IRONMAN was another challenge to move forward into. I figured I'd suck at it, so that pushed me to pursue it. I decided to train for an IRONMAN within six months and have it documented and published so that I could share my experience with others and illustrate that they could succeed in something like this too, even if they didn't necessarily have the same body type as top endurance athletes. I also wanted beginners, businessmen, mothers, and time-restrained individuals to know that they didn't have to devote 20 hours per week to this sport like a lot of other triathletes do. Most of my training is based on the input of professionals, my personal experience, and research. I've included some of the research in this book, but I also want to be authentic about exactly what my personal journey contained and provide insights based on my own experience.

When I signed up for the IRONMAN, I chose to use the race as another opportunity to raise funds for the Unique Home for Girls Orphanage in Punjab, India. In 2013, my friend and business partner, Jag Chima, had asked myself and Bani J (who is an iconic fitness celebrity in India) if we would be interested in participating in a charity event for the orphanage. Both Jag and Bani are Punjabi, so it was an appropriate fit. After that event, I visited the orphanage on several occasions and used my status and challenges to raise funds and awareness for these little girls. Many girls are abandoned as children in India because these particular parents prefer boys. Girls are abandoned in fields, dumpsters, wells, and streets. The orphanage has developed kiosks with a cot where these abandoned babies can be placed so the orphanage can better take the children in without the danger of exposed abandonment. Knowing what these girls have gone through gives me the strength of perspective to endure through pain, exhaustion, injury, doubt, and excuse. I know that if I succeed every day, I provide a possible chance for them to also succeed. The IRONMAN was another one of those opportunities to help so, no matter what, I had to finish.

FINDING A COACH

At the beginning of the process, my first thought was to wonder whether I should lose as much muscle as I could to get as light as possible and allow myself more efficiency. But I knew I would never get down to the same size as other triathletes, because I'd been weight training for 18 years and built up a level of muscle density that would take a long time to get rid of. I decided that I wanted to train for the IRONMAN without giving up my weight training or my muscle mass. I actually reached out to Dave Scott and spoke with him on the phone several times because he is an advocate of training with weights while competing as a triathlete, and he is the pro I look up to the most. I started looking to see if there was anyone who had previously done what I was aiming to do. I could find overweight people who had done it, but they only had their weight to hold them back—muscle tissue requires more oxygen, more calories, more hydration, and more blood, which is more high-stress than just weight itself.

Finally, I came across a person named Alex Viada. I remember seeing a photo of him bent over, in an aero position on a bike with an aero helmet and these massive, bulging biceps, in an IRONMAN event. I thought, *Who IS this guy?* I knew I'd found who I was looking for. He is a great coach, has a company called Complete Human Performance, and has published a book, *Hybrid Athlete*. He can deadlift over 600 pounds, yet he can run an ultramarathon—he has actually done what I wanted to achieve. I reached out to him and told him about the IRONMAN project and video series that I wanted to do. Luckily, Alex was familiar with who I was, and he was completely on board. After speaking to him, I was completely sold that this guy knew everything about the process down to the last detail. He was logical but also extremely scientific in his approach. I always say that knowledge without mileage is bullshit. Alex definitely had the knowledge, and he'd definitely put in the mileage. He was doing what I wanted to do, at a similar size, and he was teaching others to adapt one discipline to another based on carrying that sort of weight. I knew I would be able to relate to him and learn from him based on his personal experiences. We agreed to work together, and I began the process of training for a full IRONMAN. Alex helped me with my cardio strategy and technique in the three disciplines of swimming, biking, and running for the "heavier" athlete, while I designed my weight program to coincide with the cardio.

GETTING OUTSIDE BENEFITS BOTH THE BODY AND MIND

As someone who was previously a self-proclaimed gym rat, I immediately noticed some of the holistic benefits of this new training regimen. I was spending large amounts of time outside, and I was able to explore the town I'd been living in for years and see it in a new light. A study from *Environmental Health and Preventative Medicine* was published proving that spending time in nature lowers cortisol levels, pulse rate, and blood pressure, so these benefits were certainly not all in my mind.[3] I explored streets and trails by running and by bike and then the local ponds, reservoirs, and rivers during my open water swims. I discovered this whole world, and I could go explore it and enjoy it while improving my fitness at the same time. Exercise is a beautiful way to explore new places.

HOW TRAINING FOR AN IRONMAN WILL IMPROVE YOUR LIFE

It seems that there are sometimes negative perceptions toward the pursuit of fitness. People sometimes view it as a self-absorbed vanity project. But there are too many benefits for the positive results to be overlooked. It creates an outlet for stress and negative emotions, so it improves relationships with everyone, whether they

"

**KNOWLEDGE
WITHOUT MILEAGE
IS BULLSHIT.**

"

are familial relationships, romantic relationships, business rela-tionships...you're being a bit selfish in taking care of yourself, but in the long run it allows you to give more of yourself to others. You feel better about yourself, which leads to quality time with the people in your life.

Of course, too much of a good thing can be bad for you. Push-ing physical boundaries too far can lead to scarring of the heart and possible injury, but this is experienced by very few elite athletes with excessive high volume training. Triathlon training, as I see it, is very versatile. Unlike marathon runners, we are exposing ourselves to different stressors from weight training, swimming, cycling, and running—and when compounded with recovery activities such yoga, meditation, and stretching, the training can be incredibly beneficial to your health.

As I mentioned in the last chapter, there is such an environ-ment of competition and pressure surrounding team sports. With bodybuilding and triathlons, that doesn't necessarily exist as much. You don't have to be on the podium to be a winner. Personally, I wanted to finish the IRONMAN as a bodybuilder; that in itself is an achievement. I just wanted to cross the finish line, and when they said, "You're an IRONMAN," I was going to gain a lot of fulfillment. After I went to the gym and completed my workout, I could go to bed at night and think, *I succeeded at something today.* I want to have that experience every single day of my life.

If you look at the statistics of marathon running, triathlon groups, running groups, and Spartan races, they are going through the roof. And, surprisingly, the largest category is the 40-45 age group.[4] I think this statistic is partially due to the fact that, at that age, people have raised kids and life is a bit more cushioned, sched-uled, repetitive, and convenient.

However, people are dealing with depression, bipolar symp-toms, anxiety, and thoughts of suicide more so than they ever have. Maybe the convenience of our lives is working against us, because we have no physical purpose. We evolved to be out in nature and be

"

PERSONALLY, I WANTED TO FINISH THE IRONMAN AS A BODYBUILDER; THAT IN ITSELF IS AN ACHIEVEMENT.

"

active, we evolved to hunt—but there's nothing left for us to hunt. People wonder, *What's my purpose?* They want to work for something. So they sign up for a Spartan race, or a triathlon, or a marathon. These activities are the perfect drugs for these people because they make them feel alive, with positive physical benefits on the side. The sense of achievement and fulfillment that they gain can motivate them to take steps forward in other aspects of their life, as well.

As a bodybuilder, I've seen more insecurities in my industry than in any others I've experienced. I've been in it for 18 years, and it just seems to be getting worse. People compare themselves to everyone else all the time. I'll go to an expo, and beforehand everyone will be dieting down as if they're going to compete...but they're not. They're just going to visit. Bodybuilding can be so much more than a vanity project—the muscles on our frames can be just as functional as they are visual. Our bodies are the vessels that are going to carry us for our entire lives. The body is a gift equivalent to a multi-million-dollar, amazing house. Every time we make choices that negatively affect our body, we are breaking a window of that house, smashing a brick, losing the foundation. Improving our fitness and making healthy choices helps improve the house. It's putting in the electrical system, the plumbing, making sure the house is well taken care of. Taking care of our bodies is a lifelong investment that can improve quality of life immensely. Pursuing fitness for health reasons rather than vanity leads to fulfillment, and more vanity-based rewards will come secondarily. They are an automatic result of focusing on health. Exercise has provided fulfillment for me because it's helped me to beat depression and beat being overweight, and I've reversed the decline of my health. In order to be healthy, we must be functional as well—mentally healthy and balanced. Good mental health in turn leads to further positive motivation, so it's a constant constructive progression.

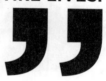

**OUR BODIES ARE THE
VESSELS THAT ARE
GOING TO CARRY US
FOR OUR ENTIRE LIVES.**

Through my pursuit of this IRONMAN, I was able to spend more time in nature and truly enjoy the process. I found that my physical, spiritual, emotional, and mental health improved right along with it. Being in gym all the time can be stifling and increase stress, but training outside, doing something completely different, has helped me to relax, create more mental space, and become more energized, focused, mentally expansive, and creative. I've found that I don't even want to run with headphones anymore, because listening to the sounds of nature and immersing myself in the experience is almost meditative. Activities like biking and swimming can be life-long sports. I hope to be swimming and cycling outside not only now, but when I'm 80 years old. A hybrid athlete training regimen leads to more balanced health, and will serve you for the rest of your life.

SECTION 2
THE BUILDING BLOCKS

CHAPTER 3
INJURY PREVENTION

When I made the decision to train for and complete a full IRONMAN, my biggest concern was injury prevention. The most common injuries triathletes sustain come from overuse, and they commonly manifest in the knee, lower leg, lower back, and shoulder.[5] My background is riddled with injuries, so I knew I was especially susceptible. I've always participated in extreme sports; I've broken bones, torn a lot of tendons, and torn a lot of muscles through motocross, downhill mountain biking, surfing, snowboarding, etc. In the early stages of training to become a hybrid athlete it is important to take injury prevention into account, particularly as a heavier athlete.

When I started researching more and speaking to people who participated in endurance sports, I was surprised to learn that more people tend to get injured during these disciplines than weight training. I thought, *Wow, are you kidding me? It's only a jog!* But there's a high amount of repetition and impact, especially for heavier people. I learned that triathletes tend to overtrain. Some put in high amounts of volume without breaking it up with tempo days

" I WAS SURPRISED TO
LEARN THAT MORE
PEOPLE TEND TO GET
INJURED DURING THESE
DISCIPLINES THAN
WEIGHT TRAINING. **"**

or recovery days. By pushing the intensity every time, they subject their bodies to a repetitive strain without recovery, which in time leads to injuries. I knew I wouldn't be putting in excessive volume, but I planned to be weight training at the same time as my cardio training for the IRONMAN, so it would be difficult for me to recover from the weight training while still putting in the necessary time for the three triathlon disciplines. I had zero background in training for swimming, cycling, or running, so I knew this would be a different training experience and I would have to be careful. I started looking up all the injuries I've had over the years, especially in my lower body and shoulders, so that I could plan how to avoid injury and be proactive from the very start of the process. There is a self-test at the end of this chapter for you to evaluate your own potential weaknesses and take an aggressive approach to injury prevention.

Staying injury-free remained a top priority, since I had decided to write this book about my experiences. If I sustained an injury in the middle of the process, I would have to quit training and everything would be put to waste. That created a lot of pressure for me to stay healthy. I was glad for the pressure, though, because it forced me to put a lot of attention into the details. A lot of the injury prevention practices I adopted are things that can be done at age 73 as well as 43 if one's smart about it. I wanted to enjoy the process of training for the race. I didn't want to drag myself over the finish line; I wanted to be present and acknowledge my achievement in the moment. Whenever I've gotten injured and had to continue my training, I cease enjoying it. Training is my therapy, so I want to make sure that it continues to be something that makes me feel good.

A BODYBUILDER'S APPROACH TO EFFICIENT RUNNING

I knew running presented the highest risk of injury since I would be sustaining the most impact, but I also knew I couldn't run on a treadmill all the time to minimize that impact; I would have to get out on the streets and the trails. In addressing my injury prevention regimen, I decided to analyze myself from the foundation up.

FEET

The feet of heavier people tend to flatten over time. Standing, walking, running, squatting, leg pressing, and performing other exercises exerts pressure onto the arches. The connective tissue in between the metatarsal bones becomes very tight, which can lead to flat feet. Sometimes it's genetic as well. But our arches are our suspension system, and since my feet were very flat, a lot of shock went through my foot and ran up through my knees, my hips, my posterior chain, and my spine. Naturally, I sought to improve the elasticity of the tissue in my feet to lessen the impact running had on the rest of my body. In the morning I rolled my feet out for three to five minutes on a tennis ball and eventually worked my way up to a golf ball.

ANKLES

I have extremely skinny ankles. I've torn the tendons in my ankles eight or nine times and broken my ankle. A few times I've rolled my feet out so fast that I've torn the internal *and* external tendons. Knowing that I'd be running on road and off road, I was concerned about how high the chances were for that injury to reoccur. I incorporated ankle exercises into my workouts: Three times per week I would do 30 rotations of my ankle in each direction and 30 flexions for several sets. I thought it was going to be easy, but after 20

> **IN ADDRESSING MY INJURY PREVENTION REGIMEN, I DECIDED TO ANALYZE MYSELF FROM THE FOUNDATION UP.**

rotations on the very first set my ankles were absolutely burning. That's when I realized how weak my ankles actually were; you might be surprised to find that yours are weaker than expected, too. I started incorporating more ankle work into my routines: I'd stand on an aero mat in the gym—a spongy mat that is difficult to balance on—and stand on one foot while slowly rotating my torso side to side. Once I mastered that, I began balancing on a BOSU Ball one foot at a time.

For the first couple weeks I couldn't balance for more than three seconds without having to put my second foot down, but I gradually began to see improvement and transitioned into doing the majority of my lower leg exercises—such as squatting, lunging, or deadlifting—with one or both feet on a BOSU ball. This technique is an unconventional approach, and looks unstable. It can be dangerous if you're not doing it correctly. I posted a couple of videos online and received some backlash because people had never seen me do anything like that before. I was known for hardcore bodybuilding movements, keeping them basic and very heavy. But as much as the haters criticized me, I started to vastly improve and there was no doubt I was onto something. When I was on the BOSU ball, the only thing stopping my ankles from snapping or rolling out was the strength of the tendons, ligaments, and connective tissue. As I was strengthening that area to prevent my feet from everting all the time on the BOSU ball, I also began strengthening my tibialis anterior using a lower cable machine. I would add some ankle weight, then pull my toes up to dorsiflex. This made a big difference. The other thing that helped was trail running, with exposure to the bumps and rocks and divots. When on the trails, you need to be fully present the whole time and focus on your foot placement. Stepping on variable terrain helps strengthen the ankles. After implementing all these strategies, I didn't feel unstable at all anymore.

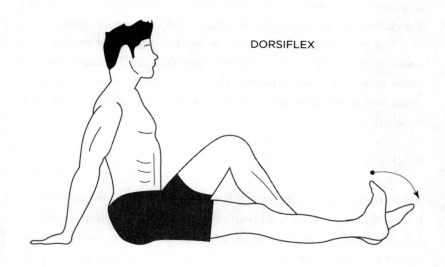
DORSIFLEX

SHIN SPLINTS

One of the most common running and triathlon injuries, for many people but especially heavier people, is shin splints. As people started following my program, one of the most common questions was, "How do I get rid of shin splints?" I used to have terrible shin splints, but I bought a roller stick and used it to roll down the muscles in my calves and my tibialis anterior a couple times per week after I ran, then I'd ice them to get rid of any inflammation. But by far, the biggest thing that helped with my shin splints was wearing the correct trainers and learning how to forefoot strike correctly. I recommend having a gait analysis done by a professional, who will test your gait and then recommend trainers that match your foot strike and shape of your foot. I purchased all three of the top trainers recommended to me, then alternated between them to avoid having the exact same point of repetitive strain on my feet the whole time.

KNEES

After I had improved the strength of my ankles, I next focused on my knees. Knees can bear the brunt of exercise for many bodybuilders. Repetitive stress while running as a heavier person, and then the added resistance we place upon them weekly within the weights room, can take its toll if not exercised correctly. I started doing movements unilaterally as opposed to bilaterally to strengthen each individual knee. I did pistol squats, lunges, leg extensions one leg at a time, and when I did lunges on the BOSU ball I made sure my knees were aligned and tracking. I began running on trails instead of hard surfaces to lessen the impact. I would train legs before some of my longer runs to pre-fatigue my leg muscles so I could justify doing much less mileage than a general triathlete, again to lessen volume impact and the likelihood of injury.

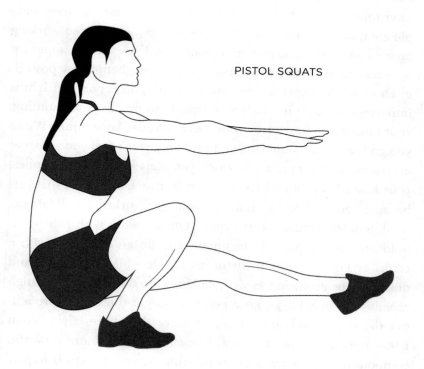

PISTOL SQUATS

LOWER BACK

The other common injury for the heavier runner is the lower back. When you run, you must hold up your upper body. When fatigue sets in, usually the first thing to go is posture. Many people will work the "mirror muscles"—the ones they can see: their chests, shoulders, and arms. But they don't focus on the muscles that aren't as visible, such as the ones in their backs. In their legs most people are quad dominant, and I was no exception. I started working on my hamstrings and posterior chain to balance out my upper leg muscles and to improve my posture. By strengthening my posterior chain it was easier to keep my torso upright. Staying upright is important because if you lean forward too much while running, your knee could travel over your toes and cause knee injury. When you go for a 3 to 6 mile run, you probably won't feel your posture deteriorating too much. But when you start hitting 8 to 12 miles, your lower back can noticeably start to tire. Don't think that just because you don't feel it initially, it won't get worked. It will fatigue.

I generally did a lot of hyperextension work with cables. I'd hold onto a low pulley attachment and do an extension with a cable, or I'd have dumbbells in my hands while coming up and doing a hype extension as well, making sure that I was doing high repetitions—maybe 30, 40 repetitions to get that burn throughout the lower back and obviously work the entire back. When I felt more stable in this area, I began targeting more powerful compound movements such as deadlifts. Core strength is hugely important, because with a heavier upper body you tire more quickly. If you start to lean forward, you'll be crushing your diaphragm, so then you can't breathe, and you fatigue even further at a dramatic rate.

"

**CORE STRENGTH IS
HUGELY IMPORTANT,
BECAUSE WITH
A HEAVIER UPPER
BODY YOU TIRE
MORE QUICKLY.**

"

SHOULDERS

The last major area I focused on for injury prevention was my shoulders. I've separated my AC joints and I've torn my infraspinatus, so I'd had a lot of shoulder problems in the past. My left shoulder was more restricted than my right, so I noticed training issues during swim workouts. My left elbow doesn't come up as high as my right, so if I tried to swim in a straight line, I gradually started to drift to the left because I couldn't pull as strongly on my left side. I started working on rotator cuff movements three times per week to make sure I was getting proper retraction within my shoulder blades. Unfortunately, my left shoulder got injured only weeks before the preparation for my IRONMAN journey began. I visited a top specialist who suggested a cortisone injection because surgery was not an option for me during this time. I took the shot (the first in my 18 years of weight training), which definitely helped for several weeks but it had soon worn off. I had no option but work around this issue and have surgery post IRONMAN.

Another injury prevention strategy I utilized, which I will further detail in the recovery section, was to make sure the muscle groups were always elasticized and there wasn't any knotting. In training for this IRONMAN, my legs took a huge pounding. Between weightlifting and the three disciplines, I found it necessary to foam roll four or five times per week after my workouts. I also received a massage once per week to remove lactic acid and any built-up scar tissue. Built-up scar tissue can have a negative effect on any movements, which over time can cause injury. I utilized heat therapy and ice therapy. I'd take a hot bath most nights, and I'd take an ice bath after hard sessions, particularly following long bike rides. Regardless of what you need to do for injury prevention, take the opportunity to turn your weaknesses into weapons.

TAKE THE OPPORTUNITY TO TURN YOUR WEAKNESSES INTO WEAPONS.

INJURY TIPS

- Your past injuries are part of your story. Don't forget about them! They may very well revisit you during this epic training experience.

- Visiting a physical therapist to assess your physiology and potential for different type of injuries could provide a huge benefit on the front end.

- Listen to your body. If it says to warm up your knees with step-ups and extensions before squats, do it.

- If you're nursing any injuries, use de-load weeks as a chance to give them space to heal.

- Injuries and equipment malfunctions happen. Deal with them! Don't let a rolled ankle or flat bike tire stop you from completing your workouts. Finish your cardio on a stationary bike or in a pool if you need to. No excuses.

SELF-TEST FOR INJURY PREVENTION

ANKLE SPRAINS

If ankle stability is a possible area of concern for you, I suggest that you check your flexibility by flexing, dorsiflexing, and rotating your ankle to the left and right to see if it triggers any discomfort or tightness in one area more than another. Take a look at the bottom of your older running trainers to see if they wear more on the outside or inside, which can indicate if you tend to pronate to the inside or outside. Depending on your rotation, you can then work the opposing side of the ankle to stabilize this area.

Although this is a self-help assessment section, you can also find a local sports shoe store or running store that offers gait analysis to better judge your gait and provide both shoe and running recommendations to correct your foot strike and form.

If you do have an ankle weakness, I suggest you begin strengthening the area with these exercises:

- Perform 30 rotations to the right, 30 to the left, and then 30 flexions and dorsiflexions for 3 sets, 3 times per week.

- Begin performing bodyweight squats and lunges upon a BOSU ball. These will feel very unstable to begin with because the connective tissue around the ankle is weak and placed in a vulnerable position. As you get stronger, the ankle will feel more stable and you will feel less vulnerable to injury in this area.

KNEE ALIGNMENT

The balance and tracking of left to right in each leg is important to keep your feet, ankles, knees, and hips safe. Here's a self-test to try for knee alignment:

Standing on one leg in front of a mirror, shift the weight to your left foot and lift your right leg, extending it in front of you. Slowly bend your left knee and lower your hips back into a pistol squat. As you do, pay close attention to where your left knee moves. Does it track to the right or left? Repeat on the other side and watch the right knee's progress.

If your self-test shows that your knee is out of track (indicating weakness), try these exercises:

- Single-leg standing balance poses on a wobble board or BOSU ball. Perform 3 sets of 1-minute balances per leg, 6 minutes in total.

- Pistol Squats. Perform 3 sets of 20 reps per leg.

If your self-test indicates inflexibility in the inner thigh (identified by spreading your legs into a split stretch then leaning forward—if you can't touch your hands to the floor you are likely very tight in your inner thigh), include these poses in your practice:

- Romanian Deadlift holding a dumbbell in each hand for resistance. Perform 3 sets of 20 reps per leg.
- Walking Lunge holding a dumbbell in each hand for resistance. Perform 3 sets of 20 reps per leg.

BACK AND CORE WEAKNESS

To test for possible future back issues, I'd advise the following:

Try walking at a slight incline over several miles. You can even wear a small backpack for added resistance. If you find that your posture begins to sag and you feel discomfort in your lower back, this is a sign of lumbar and erector isometric stability weakness. Left alone, this can lead to premature fatigue, limited respiratory function, and spinal injury.

To help condition you, I'd suggest the following:

- Good mornings. Perform 5 sets of 20 reps and do this 2-3 times per week.
- Walk/hike inclines with a weighted vest or weighted backpack. Begin with 3 miles and gradually work up to 8 miles. Focus on walking completely upright. If you can't keep your posture aligned, you have walked too far. Do this 1-3 times per week.
- Take a yoga or Pilates class 1-2 times per week. This will help you connect, engage, and strengthen your core so you can subconsciously align your posture while running and cycling in the aero position.

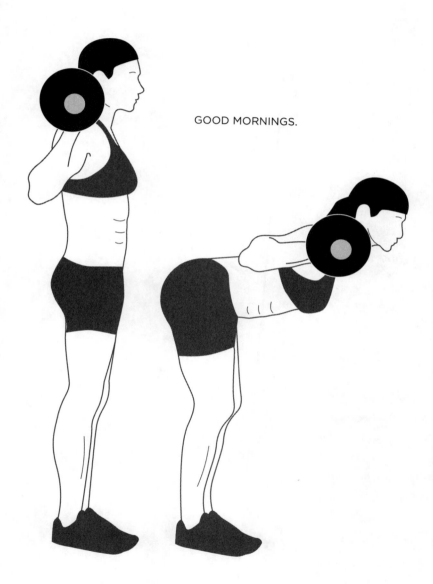

GOOD MORNINGS.

CHAPTER 4
TECHNIQUE

As I started training for the IRONMAN, I realized I couldn't even complete the necessary volume of work to build fitness because I was so unfit. I needed to learn more about technique in order to effectively train at all. As confirmed by a study from *Medicine and Science in Sports and Exercise*, correct form leads to higher energy efficiency, which will allow you to cover more ground with less effort—an important element when you're training for endurance performance.[6] Technique training was a huge aspect of the coaching I received from Alex Viada and others because it is imperative for effective triathlon training, regardless of hybrid athlete status. Although competing in an IRONMAN is an individual endeavor, it can take a team and additional knowledge markers to distinguish efficiency in your discipline. Luckily, I learned a lot from other trainers, Alex Viada, books, studies, magazines and my own efforts. You could say this book is a big part of your effort—you already have me on your team. This chapter is broken up into three sections: one each for the swim, the bike, and the run.

THE SWIM

Swimming had always been an activity I would do...if I had to. If I wiped out wake surfing, had to get across a river, or went for a dip in a hotel pool, I would swim. When I signed up for the IRONMAN, which includes a 2.4-mile swim, I knew I would have to put in a large number of yards frequently. Being a little more muscular than the average person, I quickly found swimming served as a wake-up call—and you might, too.

At the beginning I could only swim a length. My legs sunk and I had the hydrodynamics to slice through water like a pillow. I thought I could just muscle my way through it, but putting in the time wasn't going to take me to being a competent IRONMAN swimmer in only 6 months. Alex Viada taught me techniques that would be my ticket to flotation with propulsion. As I came to find out, I was completely exhausted and out of breath simply focusing on certain technique drills. Knowing this, it made even more sense not to aimlessly swim laps. Focusing on singular techniques to improve with every lap made me a better, fitter, and more efficient swimmer. I was gaining three benefits for the time investment of one.

In my training I alternated using some different devices so I could target fatigue either to my upper body or lower body for any particular workout. Some days I did drills with a kickboard, to focus on improving my kick technique and strengthening my hip flexors, while other days I held a buoy between my legs to keep them stationary and wore paddles on my hands to work my triceps and strengthen my upper body. I practiced using my legs less so I could conserve them for the following 112-mile cycle and 26.2-mile run in the actual race.

POSITION

The first thing to focus on is head position. I learned to dip my head down, because I'd always want to look ahead. I'm a little bit anxious in water so I'd want to see where I was going. By dipping your head down and looking at the bottom of the pool, you automatically pop your lower body up if you keep your legs straighter and in line with the upper body. This will create a parallel between your body toward top of the water and the bottom of the pool.

I went swimming up at a reservoir near Boise with Bailey Clifford, who used to be the nationally top-ranked triathlete for her age group. She noticed that I zigzagged all over the place while swimming, and recommended that I look up to sight every four to five strokes. But every time I looked up, my lower body would sink and I'd have to scramble to get back into position and reestablish my rhythm. Bailey pointed out that I was bringing my entire nose and mouth out of the water when I didn't need to. I just had to pop my eyes out. It was incredibly obvious, but sometimes we need to be told the obvious. As soon as I took her advice, swimming in open water became so much easier. My heavier legs were no longer sinking and I could maintain my position in the water without using extra energy.

I noticed that my legs would always come apart, especially as I would turn on my side to take a deep breath, because it's the body's natural response to counteract rotation. However, that creates drag and inefficiency with the kick, so be conscious of keeping your legs closer together. Kick from the hips instead of quads to create more power and efficiency.

ARM STROKE

I began working on raising my elbows higher and rotating my torso to guarantee that I was fully extending my reach and using my entire forearm as well as my hand to catch and pull. If you reach forward farther, you will be able to achieve a little more glide without encountering so much fatigue from the high repetition of arm strokes. This is fine for most, but bodybuilders have more muscle mass with the deltoids which leads to a greater pump and fatigue. In the pool, focus on decreasing your stroke count to save some strokes without losing too much speed. For the pull, it is important to use the back of the forearms as well as your cupped hand to catch and pull. Instead of just pulling your hand out of the water before the end of a stroke, you should actually push it back, similar to a tricep kickback at the gym. You will feel it when you're doing it correctly. Your triceps start burning, your lats start burning, and you want to pull with your back as opposed to just your arm. Pulling with your back will allow you to use your larger muscle groups, which won't fatigue as quickly as the smaller muscle groups.

As soon as I obtained a wetsuit and started practicing with it, I realized I would need to adjust my swim style. With the wetsuit being very tight across my chest and shoulders, I found that amount of tension was causing my shoulders to tire more quickly. When I adjusted my stroke to be a bit more like a windmill, instead of a pool stroke, I felt less fatigue in my deltoids. Usually, when swimming in a pool, when the hand is about to enter, the opposite arm begins to pull. You may find it easier to keep the arms almost opposite each other during the stroke to reduce the wetsuit stretch, and ease the intensity and resistance placed upon your deltoids.

THE BIKE

Unlike with swimming and running, I came from a biking background, but that background consisted of motocross racing and downhill mountain biking. Everything involved speed; nothing required the hard work of consistently pushing through my legs for hours on end. For downhill mountain biking we would race to the bottom of the hill and get picked up to go to the top. In training for

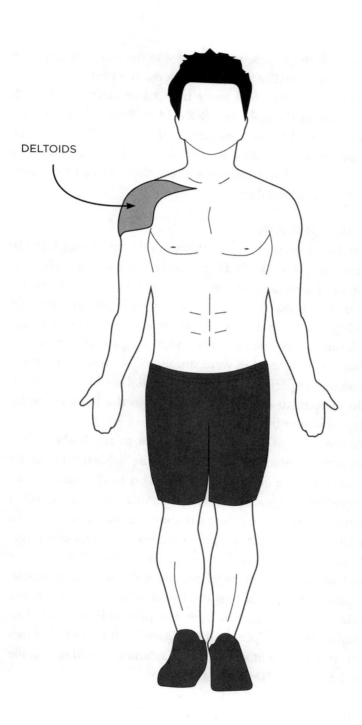

DELTOIDS

the IRONMAN, the tables turned— it was the absolute opposite of what I was used to. I've always considered road bikes to be very uncomfortable. You can feel every bump and can't go off road. It's a means to get through the IRONMAN. Mountain bikes and motorbikes are used for fun and activity. The road bike is used for an immense amount of miles. It's built for the distance. It was not my preferred form of transport out of the three bikes I just mentioned, but I learned to adapt.

SETTING UP YOUR BIKE

If you're looking to complete a triathlon or take up cycling, I highly recommend you get a bike that is the correct size for you. The correct size of the frame depends on your height. I got my bike set up at a local triathlon store called TriTown by its highly experienced owner and triathlete Antonio, who customized it for my size. Originally the frame was correct, the seat was correct, and the crank was correct, but the aero handles were simply too narrow. As a hybrid athlete, you may experience this issue as well. I could not close my arms tight enough to comfortably hold onto the handles, so he widened the aero bar handles for me.

There are a lot of equipment variables to think about, like getting an aerodynamic helmet or getting the lightest bike on the market, but those are going to be wasted on heavy athletes like myself. We're trying to just finish this thing; we're trying to continue as a bodybuilder. If we were worried about the weight of the bike and that level of aerodynamics, then we bodybuilders could just lose five pounds off our own frames in a week instead of spending a thousand dollars on a lighter wheel. But we're not losing muscle. We are hybrid athletes—so just deal with what you've got. Some people take too much time on their equipment. Hard work first, consistency second, equipment third. Dave Scott and Mark Allen didn't have the equipment as they do today, and they still have some of the top times in IRONMAN history.

On a bike, the aero position can initially feel awkward or uncomfortable, especially if you have a larger torso and larger legs because they tend to crush your diaphragm as you're pedaling. The seat felt too high at the beginning, so I began with the seat a bit lower than it should have been for a true aero position. But, after about six weeks, I started to feel comfortable and wanted move my seat up a bit so I could bring my hamstrings further into the peddling movement. Your seat height might change a few times throughout the program as you become more experienced, comfortable, and attuned with your body/bike connection. Speaking of aerodynamics, having wider and heavier frame emulates something like a sail—not good when trying to slice through the air. I try to tuck myself in to make myself as narrow and compact as possible. I also noticed that my hands would become numb if I allowed my bodyweight to push too far forward, but leaning my forearms into the aero bars (more than the lighter rider would) helped immensely.

PEDALING

Much like we all assume that we know how to walk and run, we assume we know how to ride a bike. Or pedal, at least, but that's not the case. Wearing clip-in bike shoes isn't just for looking cool—it's to enable the maximization of each pedal stroke. When you push down on the pedal, the quad is the primary muscle being used. But if you're going up a hill and you're just pushing and pushing, eventually your muscular quads are going to give out. More muscle fibers require more oxygen, energy, and blood, and produce more waste products such as lactic acid. It's necessary to distribute that intensity and fatigue throughout the hamstrings and glutes, because that's where a lot of the rotation and momentum is going to come from.

They're large muscle groups and can do a lot of the work. When I began cycling with clip-on shoes, it took me a while to figure out the correct rhythm and force to use. If you pull too much or

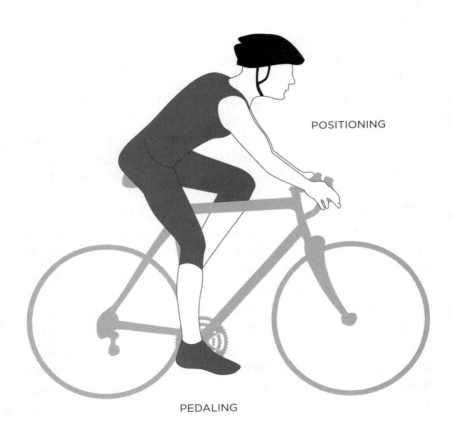

POSITIONING

PEDALING

push too much you waste extra energy, so it is key to learn to exert consistent force and stay within the realm of your crank size. If you don't, you'll be giving up about 20 percent of the power of each pedal stroke. In the gym lifting weights, your muscles engage, then disengage—but on the bike they must be engaged, even just a little, the whole time.

POSITIONING

When it came to cycling technique, the primary aspect I needed to improve was my knee position. My knees frequently splayed out as I would pedal to avoid hitting my torso, and when I saw videos of myself I thought, *What am I doing?* I looked like I was driving Miss Daisy with a basket on front. The position wasn't healthy for my knees and certainly not very aerodynamic. I worked on bringing my knees in closer, which wasn't easy. It placed more stress on the abductor and flexor muscles and caused them to fatigue more quickly, but it started to get easier and paid off in efficiency. If this doesn't work for you, you can look at getting a slightly shorter crank to accommodate the quad-to-torso contact. Have an experienced cyclist watch you, or film yourself to look at your pedal movements and identify areas of improvement.

I also found that while pedaling, I used my upper body automatically to twist into the movement. When cycling, focus on keeping as still as possible, which exerts less energy and makes it easier to breathe. Spending long amounts of time in the aero position can cause the triceps and core to tire and become uncomfortable. To counter this effect, I started to do planks after my workouts in the gym, whether on the floor or a Swiss ball. It created more stability and balance in my core, as well as getting quite uncomfortable after a certain amount of time. Learn to get comfortable being uncomfortable—I recommend doing a lot of planks so your body will be used to that kind of fatigue on the bike.

" LEARN TO GET COMFORTABLE BEING UNCOMFORTABLE. "

HILLS

When it comes to hills, the bigger athlete is going to have a lot of trouble. We use 6 watts of extra power per kilogram of body weight if we're on as little as a 2 percent gradient. Heavier and more muscular athletes must be aware that we're going to go through many more calories, a lot of power, and overexert very quickly on hills if we don't hold back. It's very easy for us to run out of energy, in which case we won't be able to continue biking. I had to be comfortable easing up and going slow, allowing lighter people to overtake me, because they find it so much easier. Mentally I needed to be okay with that. Remember, you can take advantage of your weight on the flat road and the decline. Up to 30 percent of additional energy is used standing up when going uphill, and again, with more muscle on the frame, there is a lot of weight to carry. As much as I wanted to get competitive and stand up, I forced myself to sit down to conserve energy. At TriTown they recommended some of their athletes not to go over 220 watts of power on an incline...on an incline, if I was to do 220 watts I'd probably bike 1 mile per hour and fall on my side. When I rode with other triathletes on hills I would usually ask their wattage. If they were on 200, I was usually around 330, maybe 350 watts just because of my size and weight.

Exercises such as squats, leg press, lunges and deadlifts had made my legs very powerful but they weren't trained to sustain the large amount of reps by pushing down on the pedals time and time again. I needed to transition my years of Type 2 fast twitch muscle fiber training to the more sustained Type 1 slow twitch muscle fiber recruitment via higher reps, and increasingly sustained cycling efforts.

A steady pace is the only way to successfully compete over the course of the entire 112-mile ride in only 6 months prep on minimal training and as a bodybuilder. By far, the most effective way to improve hill performance is hill repeats. Find a bad hill and keep riding it. It's terrible, it's tough, it's disgusting, it's horrible, but it will lead to major improvement. Biking hills can be a mental game. To begin with, especially if you bike with other people, you're going to feel really insecure and inferior—or at least I did. You have to be comfortable with being bad at something—the worse you are, the more ground you have to make up, and the more improvements you're going to see.

ADDITIONAL EQUIPMENT

Many triathletes and cyclists, including myself, used a machine called a watt bike to train on indoors. This is a great piece of machinery. On the screen you can see the wattage of how much power you're putting out on your right leg in comparison to the power from your left leg. I noticed my left leg wasn't putting out as much complete rotational power as my right, so sometimes I would do drills where I'd just work with my left leg, and then alternate and work on the right. Just as you can alternate with a dumbbell as opposed to a barbell, efficiently focusing that force upon those muscle groups creates more neuro-muscular power and educational process to each particular muscle.

THE RUN

Being a heavier athlete, I knew the run would present the highest risk for injury and that technique was especially important. I studied the technique of a lot of top triathletes and runners to see what they were doing.

FOOT STRIKE

One of the most important techniques I adapted was the forefoot strike. Using a forefoot strike with every stride rather than a heel strike is absolutely imperative for efficient jogging, especially at my weight. This means initially landing on the balls of the feet with each stride before allowing the feet to flatten. If you were to heel strike, which means letting your heel touch the ground first, it would put significantly more stress through your ankles, shins,

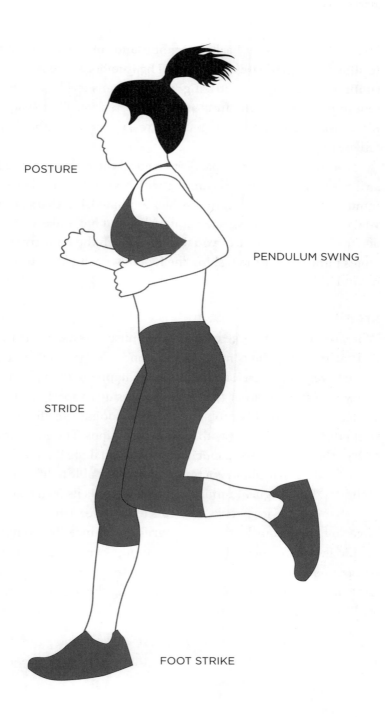

POSTURE

PENDULUM SWING

STRIDE

FOOT STRIKE

knees, hips, and lower back. Over thousands of steps this can lead to shin splints and stress fractures. The forefoot strike is not to be confused with "tip toe" striking, which means striding from one foot to the other on the front portion of the foot. Tip toe striking places way too much stress on the calves, which will either lead to fatigue or injury.

A strategy to lessen impact is to control the cadence of the foot strike. An ideal cadence is running with about 180 foot strikes per minute. It looks slightly cartoonish or animated, but that's because you're no longer running like a square box but more like a wheel. It lessens impact and causes you to pull up with the hamstrings and glutes rather than just crashing the foot down with all your weight behind it.

STRIDE

When someone has large quantities of muscle tissue in the thighs and calves, he or she is much more prone to experiencing fatigue in the lower half when jogging. Once this happens, the natural tendency is to shuffle rather than pick the legs up properly with each stride. To help fix this problem, I suggest doing specific work to strengthen the hip flexors with leg raise variations. The goal is to disengage the abdominals as much as possible, making it a specific exercise for the hip flexors. As a result, you will be able to lift your legs higher as they fatigue. Running off road presents its own challenges with roots, crevices, rocks, and ruts to run over, which naturally force you to lift your legs even higher for clearance. To strengthen the hip flexors further, whilst road running I occasionally ran with 5-10-pound weights on each ankle. Within the gym I would perform hanging and lying leg raises by disengaging the abs but engaging my hip flexors.

POSTURE

Make sure you are keeping your head aligned and looking ahead. Just like swimming, if your head is misaligned, then your posture will fall as well. One thing for posture that really helps in addition to the gym exercises I mentioned is wearing a weights vest. It can add lot of impact on the knees, but can make a positive difference if you run more off road, or even just by wearing it when going for a walk. If anything is going to cause your posture to collapse, it's the weight of that vest. Keep in mind that you must work your way up in weight gradually. To begin with I just did it on my curved treadmill, which I will discuss in the next section.

Stay conscientious of your arm position and keep your arms close to your body to conserve energy. I noticed in videos that my arms were way out, so I created a mental cue for myself to keep them in place. I'd wear a belt around my waist with two drink bottles on every run. Even if I wasn't going to drink much, I still wore the belt because I figured, if I was going to wear it in the race, I might as well get used to it as soon as possible. I knew if my arms started hitting the bottles then I was starting to fatigue and needed to pull my arms up and keep them tight to my sides. I also noticed after about five miles that my muscular dense arms would start fatiguing after holding them in a fixed position for so long, so sometimes I would switch my ankle weights to my wrists for added strength and conditioning to these areas. My arms would fatigue quickly but over time they begun to condition themselves with added strength. Soon, running without the weights was relatively easy, so I could go over double the running distance without fatigue.

PENDULUM SWING

The Pendulum Swing incorporation made a *huge* difference for me, like night and day. In Kevin Everett's book *The Heart of Running* he discusses a technique he calls the "pendulum swing." Prior to reading his book I would attempt to muscle my way through a run pumping my arms back and forth. Kevin suggests to allow the natural rotation of your hips, core, and arms to power the run to allow for optimal timing and balance. Your right foot, left hip, and right shoulder move in sync while your left foot, right hip, and left shoulder activate together with opposite timing. This pendulum rotates around an invisible sphere situated in your stomach. I found that using this twist as I ran allowed me to more fully extend from my hip, enabling me to reach my forward and backward strides farther without heel striking. I'd always think, exactly how he described, of having a sphere inside my stomach. If I tilted to one side, it would fall out. If my posture fell forward, it would fall out. As we fatigue, the diaphragm closes and we find it harder to breathe, so we fatigue even more and slow down. By thinking about keeping the sphere in place, I wasn't swaying side to side. I was keeping completely aligned, which placed less impact on the lower back and heart and lungs.

ADDITIONAL EQUIPMENT

Not everyone is going to invest in his or her own treadmill, but one piece of machinery that was fantastic for me to begin the training process was the Woodway Curve. It is a curved treadmill powered solely by your body's power and momentum. These treadmills are 30 percent more difficult than standard treadmills. I knew that, with my knees and ankles and heel strike, I was going to have a lot of problems training for the run. The beauty of the Woodway Curve is that you use your hamstrings and glutes to pull, and experience no impact through your heels because you're running on a slope. It was the perfect way to start with the weights vest because it was less impact, didn't allow quad dominance, and necessitated use of the forefoot strike. It provided me with frequent exhausting experiences with no impact upon my joints, and can be an excellent tool for someone who carries more muscle mass.

HILLS

Similar to the bike portion, when running uphill with a physique of a bodybuilder, we're going utilize so much more energy, calories, hydration, and wattage than smaller athletes. When going up a hill it's helpful to increase your cadence even more, so you are taking baby steps. Each larger stride will take a lot more exertion. It's going to be the difference of going up stairs and taking two steps at a time versus taking one step—much better going off a little bit slower and taking one step as opposed to spending the energy for two steps. Push through the toes and tilt the hips forward slightly. It will enable you to use the momentum of your weight to get you up that hill more efficiently. You can use your weight on the downhills and really make up ground there, but make sure to utilize proper downhill running technique. Keep your hips aligned perpendicular to the ground and make sure to pick up your feet behind you to lessen the impact on your joints. Relax the shoulders, strike with the whole foot, don't brake too hard but don't push yourself too hard either. Keep shoulders back, torso tight, and take small steps with a fast cadence. A little bit of achy pain in the knees is okay because it can take up to a couple of years to build up the connective tissue strength for a heavier athlete doing downhill running. After a couple years, the aches will disappear.

The hybrid athlete Cameron Hanes was very influential for me from a trail running perspective. He's a muscular athlete who often competes in ultramarathons. He runs and weight trains almost daily to be better at his career—that of a professional bow hunter. He once competed in ultramarathons at a much lighter bodyweight, but found that he struggled as a hunter when packing out the meat and carrying it back over long distances. He simply didn't have the muscle to facilitate the gathering after he had completed the hunt. He used weight training to his advantage and gained a significant amount of muscle to improve at his sporting career, while also coexisting as top competitive ultramarathon runner. He is by far the most muscular guy I have seen at the top of his sport, proving that muscle can help and not hinder progress for distance runners.

He has since inspired thousands of people, including me, to trail run. The softer, uneven surfaces are much more forgiving for the heavier athlete than typical roads and sidewalks. Harder surfaces can lead to faster wear, tear, and injury. Cameron has pushed me to use trail running in all seasons as a means to harden up and condition my resolve, all while acknowledging the meditational space with nature.

Throughout the training process, I learned about technique from a variety of sources. I read many books and articles regarding the three disciplines, but I always took their advice with a grain of salt. Techniques and programs that work for a 160-pound athlete may not work for someone of my size. Alex Viada instructed me on some of the finer points of adjusting triathlon training for a heavier muscled person. I also had conversations with other experienced triathletes, like six-time IRONMAN World Champion Dave Scott and a local top triathlete named Kenny McDaniel to gain their insights and get as much feedback as possible, which helped immensely, probably more than they know.

What my research boiled down to at the end was mostly trial and error. I noticed my own weak spots and looked into them. If I tried a technique and it led to my improvement, I stuck with it. If not, I adopted something new. There's only so much you can listen to, absorb, apply—it either works or it doesn't. You either debunk it, or you put it in your pocket and run with it. Don't look for a standard; set it.

TECHNIQUE TIPS

- Equipment that fits properly can make the difference between finishing feeling okay, and finishing in serious discomfort. Seek out specialists and get fitted!

- Bike shorts exist for a very good reason: their padded butt. If you're spending serious hours in the saddle, get over your self-consciousness and wear them!

- Swimming is just like swinging a golf club. You have to keep getting a feel for it. Keep chasing that "relaxed and efficient" feeling in the water, and it'll do more for you than chasing numbers ever does.

- Mountain biking and trail running make it tougher initially to train, but help with agility, core muscles, reaction time, and strengthening up all the protective secondary muscles. After putting in time off road, the road seems much easier.

- When doing runs, include a couple of faster-paced sections of a few hundred yards at a time, especially if you largely train on flat ground. This can help simulate the changes in elevation on a race course, or the pushes you must make to overtake someone. It is essential to mix intensity, hill, and tempo runs to target the fast-twitch muscle fibers.

ABOVE AND BEYOND

Anyone can follow the technique guidelines I've outlined in this chapter without extra equipment, but if you'd like to go above and beyond in your training there are a few higher-level options you can pursue. Continuing to educate yourself can do nothing but help you. I compiled a list of books and resources I interacted with during my training process, which is at the end of this book to provide additional references for you if you are interested in learning more.

First and foremost, gait analysis done by a professional will analyze how your body moves while running. Computer data and measurement reports can provide in-depth insights into how to improve your performance and prevent injuries. Many running stores and professionals provide this service.

Another training option, VO2 max testing, identifies the highest amount of oxygen your body can utilize during maximal exercise. During this test, you are typically hooked up to a treadmill with a breathing mask on and they measure your oxygen consumption as you work up to your peak effort level. VO2 max is a great measurement of running fitness, and can provide a tangible number to consider for pacing during running workouts.

I found two pieces of equipment to be especially helpful: my GPS watch and a power meter for my bike. Obtaining a GPS watch, such as a Garmin, can provide concrete numbers to track your performance. I am very motivated by numbers, so wearing a Garmin helped me track my training and added an extra layer of workout motivation. Platforms such as Strava allows athletes to compare their workouts with other Strava users in the area and discover new routes.

Attaching a power meter to your bike will allow you to measure your FTP (Functional Threshold Power). FTP is measured in watts and identifies your average power output over the course of an hour on the bike. Testing your FTP regularly is a great way to measure progress; even if you don't test for FTP often, a power meter will help you manage your desired effort levels during training.

CHAPTER 5
WEIGHTLIFTING

Many people, when they think about bodybuilding and working out in a gym, think about the number of weights being lifted and the aesthetics of it. But really, it's so much more than what people think it is. It can prolong and lead to a higher quality of life. Your body is built to be versatile; it is built to move and be functional. You'll be able to better assimilate food, which then can better fuel your heart, the blood flow to your brain, etc.

Bodybuilding is about building your confidence, increasing your energy, and building your bone density. It gives you an endorphin release—it makes you feel good. It's becoming more of a suggestion in hospitals and prisons to exercise. It helps people both physically and mentally. It can be a preventative measure against depression, anxiety, heart disease, or high cholesterol. There's a lot more to bodybuilding than what meets the naked eye.

I NOW PRONOUNCE YOU MUSCLE AND ENDURANCE

Many endurance athletes have an aversion to weight training because they think it will take away from their endurance training or cause them to "bulk up." For example, let's talk about the runner. They're out there training all the time, but their skeleton may not be as aligned as it should be because their muscles have atrophied. Even though they're very efficient at what they're doing, they should be strengthening their connective tissue and the muscles that surround the skeleton. That will help with postural issues, joint issues, and lead to even higher efficiency. Weight-bearing exercises improve bone density much better than drinking calcium.

Weight training leads to explosiveness, as well. If you're biking or running up a hill, or sprinting, then you need to work on your fast-twitch muscle fibers. Endurance athletes work their slow-twitch muscle fibers often, but not fast-twitch. Strength training will help engage fast-twitch. It will condition your muscles to deal with the lactate build-up of sprinting at the beginning of the race, which helps with positioning.

Weight training also helps with injury prevention for endurance athletes. If they do something outside the realm of their normal exercises for slow-twitch muscle fibers, their bodies may not be equipped to handle it and they may pull or tear their fast-twitch fibers. Your body will be altogether more functional. It feels good to be both an endurance and strength athlete. You'll be a better overall athlete. The two worlds can coexist—in the world of the hybrid athlete.

Historically, my weight workouts were extremely heavy with a lot of volume. I conventionally went for compound movements, which are exercises that use secondary muscle groups. We're talking the bench press, the deadlift, the squat, the leg press...your orthodox meat-and-potato exercises. In my transition to becoming a hybrid athlete, I knew my weights routine would have to change.

" IT FEELS GOOD TO BE BOTH AN ENDURANCE AND STRENGTH ATHLETE. YOU'LL BE A BETTER OVERALL ATHLETE. THE TWO WORLDS CAN COEXIST—IN THE WORLD OF THE HYBRID ATHLETE. "

MY UNIQUE APPROACH TO TRI TRAINING

As I mentioned in the technique chapter, I knew I had some weaknesses within the three triathlon disciplines that I could help address in the weight room.

My first priority was to incorporate unilateral exercises—one leg at a time, one side of my back at a time, one pectoral at a time—because I knew I would be unilaterally activating and deactivating those muscles during my swim, bike, and run. The goal was to mimic my training outside of the gym within the gym and customize weight training to my specific needs and weaknesses. Instead of doing traditional squats, I started doing pistol squats on one leg. If I planned to deadlift, I would do the Romanian deadlift, which works one leg at a time. I still included bilateral exercises, but unilaterally I was putting my muscles under stress in a way that would help them adapt to the new environment I was placing them in during the three disciplines.

I started working out with pieces of gym equipment that I used to laugh at people for using, such as the Swiss ball, medicine ball, aero mat, and TRX bands. I started doing many plyometric exercises I would have never done before, because I realized how important it was to work on my stability, balance, and core strength. I had to put adjustments and customizations into different parts of my weight routine, first as a triathlete and second as a heavier triathlete.

When I first started the program, I could feel weakness in my lower back while running, which indicated I needed to work on core strength. I knew my ankles were weak, so I began doing lunges and squats on a BOSU ball. In between sets I would do ankle rotations to work on my tibialis anterior, which I'd never worked before, because after a while I wouldn't be able to pick up my toes on runs.

When swimming, especially with a wetsuit on, my rotator cuffs felt extremely weak and my deltoids would burn like they'd

ROMANIAN DEADLIFT

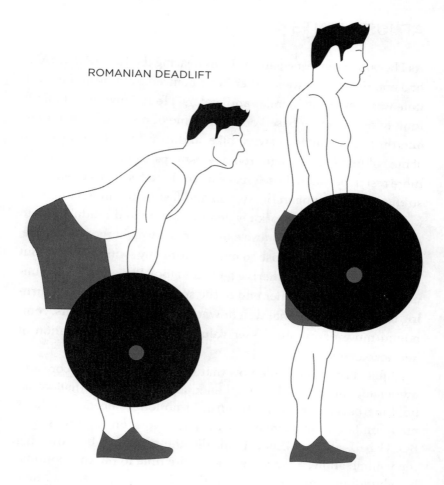

never burned before. So in the weight room I'd work with higher repetitions and work the rotator cuffs with internal and external rotation—not generally part of a traditional bodybuilder's program.

ADJUSTMENTS

As I became fitter, especially as I was nearing the Half-IRONMAN I had entered only 14 weeks after I commenced training and my volume was increasing in miles and meters, I found myself just on the limit of overtraining based on the volume of my weights workouts and three disciplines of swim, bike, and run. I had to bring down some volume in the weight room—less reps, same amount of sets, more rest in between those sets—so I could focus all my energy and strength into my anaerobic system and fast-twitch muscle fibers. I knew I didn't need to work my aerobic system and I didn't have to tap into my slow-twitch muscle fibers in the weight room anymore, because I was hitting those so much during my swim/bike/run. But I didn't want to start withering away and look like a marathon runner, so I went to the other end of the spectrum and started returning to more conventional weight workouts with free weights, compound movements, and lesser volume with the incorporation of heavier weights.

I felt very comfortable now that I'd strengthened my core and my fixator muscles. I'd strengthened any weaknesses that would hold me back in the swim/bike/run. I no longer needed to do as many unilateral movements or as much work on the Swiss ball, BOSU ball, and aero mat. I still did the exercises, but lowering the volume allowed me to dedicate more time to my conventional bodybuilding exercises such as the deadlift, bench press, and heavy curls, etc. Since I had reached so much volume in my training of the three disciplines at that point—such as a 100-mile bike ride, a 12-mile run, and a 3,000-meter swim, I brought down the volume of my weights reps but did them much, much heavier. This strategy allowed me to just tap into my type-one muscle fibers and hit

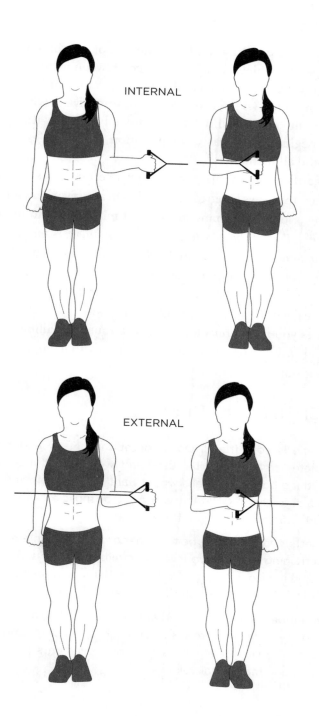

INTERNAL

EXTERNAL

my anaerobic system, then focus the rest of my time on recovery. I managed to achieve a happy balance between my different types of training, but it took trial and error. Listen to your body and give it what it wants while also making sure to give it what it needs. There is no way I could have completely written this program before beginning; it was an exploration and a series of experiments and adjustments.

Regardless of what is planned for a certain day's training, it's important to always listen to your body. On any given day, if I've been traveling a lot and in many meetings, I might think to myself, *You know what, I'm not going to deadlift today. I'll still work my back, but I'll stick to mainly machines because I feel dehydrated and I don't feel rested, so I may not warm up properly.* I know I will have less chance of injury and be able to complete my training most effectively by adapting to the given situation. If you go to a gym you're not used to, or the machines you need aren't available, you must be willing to change things up a bit. Complete similar exercises that target the same muscle groups.

WEIGHTLIFTING TIPS

- Muscle is your friend. Don't forget that! Many endurance athletes treat it like it's just dead weight, but muscle is anything but dead. That's what I want to show you. You can complete this IRONMAN with a lot of muscle, with much more efficiency than you think.

- Whether you're a pure bodybuilder or a hybrid athlete, your leg training is where your real commitment shows. A lot of people miss out on legs. So this is what separates the men from the boys...it's just short term pain.

- Remember, when compound exercises are on the menu, you need fewer total exercises since each one works so many muscles and joints. When it's isolation movements, use more moves and more total volume.

- Struggling to fit all the cardio into a single day? Split it up as necessary. 45-60 minutes in the morning and another 45-60 minutes in the evening can produce incredible results over a two-hour single session.

- If you're training for an epic endurance event, at some point you'll have to dial back the volume of strength training. Embrace it, or you'll end up under-recovered and ripe for injury.

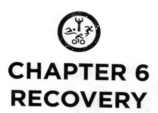

CHAPTER 6
RECOVERY

Alex Viada's words of wisdom ring true: "Get aggressive about recovery." Some days will be hard, and other days will be very, very easy. Expect it, and don't hang out too much in that tweener zone where it's not hard enough to push your limits, but too hard to easily recover from. If you haven't already, start getting serious about recovery. Take a hot bath. Take an ice bath. Get a massage, foam roll, take plenty of antioxidants, eat or supplement with protein at every meal, and don't take in anything that will give your stomach an inflammatory response such as unhealthy foods. This shit is real! Track everything, and figure out what you could be doing better.

SLEEP

They say that the standard amount of sleep needed to recover is eight hours, but it really depends for every person. Maybe you need more than eight hours. If you sleep five to six hours and you can function, recover, and are in great health, then maybe you're recovering more efficiently, your protein synthesis is higher, and you're absorbing the nutrients you need to.

"IF YOU HAVEN'T ALREADY, START GETTING SERIOUS ABOUT RECOVERY."

Do what works for you. Some people function well when they take naps, some don't. Personally, having grown up on the farm and taken on many extra jobs, I am unable to take naps. During the day I can't switch my brain off and, if I do sleep during the day, it takes me hours to fully wake up and get my brain going again.

Many people ask me, "What can I do to help me sleep?" Before I suggest anything, I recommend taking a blood test. Some people take melatonin, but their serotonin and dopamine levels are off. They can take all the 5-HTP supplements in the world, but it's not going to help them if they haven't fixed their hormonal response.

Melatonin does help some people sleep more deeply, but the main thing I suggest is to always empty your brain before going to bed. If you need to meditate in the evening, it may take a couple of months before you're able to switch off. Don't think you've been doing something for years and you're going to start meditating and it will be fine. In bodybuilding, you're not going to look like a top bodybuilder after a couple of years. You must do the boring, monotonous, foundational work first, then you might see some success from it. It's the same with meditation—it will take a while to break down the wiring that is making us wired and tired in the evening.

Some of my personal strategies include getting rid of any standby lights in the room, making sure the curtains are completely blacked out, keeping the windows open for fresh air as opposed to air conditioning, and making sure the temperature is relatively cool. Routine is important. Before I go to bed I will switch off all electrical components to prevent any blue light messing with my brain, then I'll read for about thirty minutes or so, which normally puts me right to sleep. Do not take your phone into your bedroom. Keep it in another room. If it's your alarm, I suggest you get an alarm clock. Research shows that the childhood obesity epidemic is worsened by kids taking their phones to bed, because the blue light prevents them from sleeping as much as they should be and they're not burning and storing calories when they're supposed to be.[7]

If you need to drink water during the night, keep it in your room so you don't have to go downstairs and be exposed to the light of the fridge and habit of getting up.

NUTRITION AND SUPPLEMENTATION

As I will address in later chapters, nutrition and supplementation play a massive role in recovery. Endurance sports and heavy weight-lifting put high amounts of stress on the body, leading to high cortisol levels and free radical damage. And when you push your body to the limit, micro tears are created in your muscles. To counteract this damage and repair those tears, it's extremely important to consume the proper balance of protein, vitamins, minerals, and antioxidants. It's not about what you eat; it's about what you absorb. That's what helps you recover. I have a detox drink every morning and undergo colonic hydrotherapy every week to make sure my insides are completely clean and able to absorb every nutrient I put inside my body.

Make sure the majority of your food is protein-based to assist in repairing muscle fibers after you break them down during exercise. Consuming glutamine and BCAA supplements will feed your muscles with amino acids. The faster your muscles absorb those amino acids, the faster you will recover from hard workouts. Hydration is also a key element of recovery—our bodies are made of 70 percent water, and proper hydration transports nutrients to where your body needs them.

MENTAL RECOVERY

When I was living in India, I was going through a bad time personally. I was very angry, and to an extent I thought it was a good thing, because that anger fueled me to work harder and train harder. But eventually I realized that, though I had convinced myself anger worked for me, I wasn't happy. I had lost sight of what success meant. Success isn't materialistic; it comes in some form of happiness. At that point I started looking into meditation, but I found it didn't really work for me. I worked with a few teachers, but I couldn't just lie down and switch off. I couldn't focus on my breath and the blood flow to my fingers and that sort of traditional stuff. I quickly realized I needed active meditation. I began paddle boarding, painting, and going to yoga. I even started a band for a little while and put out an album. I found that a form of active meditation—anything besides work or training that would allow me to concentrate on something I enjoyed and could relax doing—allowed me to switch off and clean my slate.

It's taken a couple of years, but now I feel that I'm actually in the place where I can lie down on a bed in a quiet room and succeed in relaxation meditation. If you can't achieve conventional relaxation meditation, look into some sort of activity and focus on your own thoughts during that activity. Remind yourself what you should be grateful for. When you reiterate that on a daily basis, you feel more at ease with yourself and are able to focus on what you want to attain. Meditation is only going to have a positive effect on your cortisol levels—which are obviously through the roof when you're on this program—and we're doing everything we can to lower them.

RECOVERY TIPS

- When you can read a book for 15 minutes in an ice bath... you're officially a badass.

- With the amount of volume in the training plan at certain junctures, it's crucial to make rest and recovery a higher priority. Completely rest when you're not training. If you have a laborious job, take that into account.

- Always get some exercise and workouts in after a flight. Along with hydration, it's a crucial way of recovering from the rigors of travel. Even just a powerwalk on the treadmill can be a lifesaver from jetlag. I also supplement with KAGED MUSCLE Citrulline to better improve my blood flow when in the pressurized cabins of planes.

- Maximize your passive recovery, not just active recovery. That means ice baths, massage, rest, and nailing your nutrition.

CHAPTER 7
NUTRITION

Training for a triathlon burns an incredible amount of calories. When creating my nutrition program, I needed to make sure I was consuming enough healthy food to fuel my swimming, biking, and running workouts while still building muscle from my bodybuilding workouts. I put 100 percent focus into not only my physical training plan, but my nutrition plan also. The goal was to look like a bodybuilder and function like a triathlete. This style of training only works if you eat, supplement, and hydrate adequately. If you don't take in enough fuel, you won't make it.

More muscular athletes have more powerful engines, like those of a Mustang or a Ferrari. Ferraris run out of gas quickly if you push them hard. A more fuel-efficient car may not be as powerful but it will travel farther. An IRONMAN is geared toward distance, so you must be careful not to run out of fuel too soon. When you start hitting the hills, if you run out of energy, you won't be able to just stop at a gas station, refuel, and return to the same level of performance.

For most of each week, I followed the nutritional guidelines and calculations based on my 12-week muscle building program. My nutritional plan includes a variety of proteins, carbohydrates, healthy fats, fruits, and some dairy. This variety is included to fuel muscle

" MORE MUSCULAR ATHLETES HAVE MORE POWERFUL ENGINES, LIKE THOSE OF A MUSTANG OR A FERRARI. FERRARIS RUN OUT OF GAS QUICKLY IF YOU PUSH THEM HARD. "

growth, power diverse workouts, and help with recovery from the two-headed assault of the weight room and sport-specific training. You must look at every single micronutrient, macronutrient, and antioxidant as having some purpose, whether it be repairing free radical damage, repairing muscle tissue, fueling the workout, or recovering from the last one. I created more detail in this program than any other nutrition plan I've created in the past because this program is placing more demand on the body—I'm trying to recover from several different types of activity and perform at the same time, as a bigger person.

Not only does nutrition contribute to recovery, it also bolsters the immune system. About four months into the training process, I started to get sick. I hadn't been sick in a few years, and it was no coincidence that I started feeling worse. My body was so busy trying to recover all the time, it didn't have time to build and maintain a very strong immune system. Cardio isn't too strenuous on the central nervous system, but weight training is. In a normal situation like this, I would have backed off the weight training for a week to give my body time to bounce back. But since I had such limited time to progress to the necessary point for the IRONMAN and was shooting the MAN of IRON video series in tandem, I didn't have that luxury. To a certain degree it was necessary for me to over-train a bit. Being aware of the situation, I over-emphasized certain antioxidants and micronutrients. I upped my intake of Zinc, Vitamin C with bioflavonoids, Echinacea, fermented glutamine, garlic, turmeric, fermented BCAAs, Re-Kaged, and lemon. Knowing that, in this case, sickness is likely from the rigors of how hard you are pushing yourself, taking these vitamins and supplements should be a preventative measure than a reactionary treatment. It's important to stay on top of your nutrient ratio. Even if you intake an overload of vitamins and minerals, as long as they are water-soluble your body will automatically flush out the excess and you'll be no worse for the wear.

Extreme endurance athletes, on average, tend to have a shorter lifespan than other athletes, which is counterintuitive, but it's because of the extreme sustained damage they are doing to their bodies over a number of years. Endurance athletes build up a huge amount of free radical damage within their bodies based on their cortisol levels going up and sustaining, along with the high levels of oxygen they intake over a prolonged period of time. Sometimes scarring to the heart has led to this contributing factor. To counteract this damage, it's extremely important to consume and absorb enough antioxidants. I want to make sure this nutrition plan creates longevity. It's not just the number of calories you consume, it's the form of the calories and the nutritional benefits they provide your body. This is not a weight-loss plan; it's a muscle-building and performance plan. To get started on the nutrition plan, use the formula below.

Nutrition formula:

Consume 1.5 grams of protein per pound of bodyweight.
Consume 2.5 grams of carbs per pound of bodyweight.
Consume 0.55 grams of fats per pound of bodyweight.

This formula will provide specific numbers to establish your calorie and macronutrient intake during the MAN of IRON program based on your body weight.

You'll be consuming six meals per day. This nutrition plan is different than those for the typical triathlete. It's higher in protein to recover and maintain muscle mass. Heavier athletes utilize significantly more proteins, carbohydrates, vitamins, and antioxidants. Your body doesn't produce certain nutrients that you'll need to supplement your diet. Be warned: Your body will be screaming for calories both good and bad, and you'll need to keep stuffing only good ones into it until it finally shuts up. There are no cheat meals on this plan, but you'll eat well enough and often enough that you won't need one.

BE WARNED: YOUR BODY WILL BE SCREAMING FOR CALORIES BOTH GOOD AND BAD, AND YOU'LL NEED TO KEEP STUFFING ONLY GOOD ONES INTO IT UNTIL IT FINALLY SHUTS UP.

PROTEIN SOURCES

Proteins will provide the amino acids necessary to recover and build muscle tissue. It's important to stick to lean sources of protein so as not to take in unnecessary fat. Pouring extra egg whites on top of your fried, whole eggs in the pan is an easy way to boost protein content. An even easier way is to drink a KAGED MUSCLE Protein Shake.

Sources of lean protein:

- Salmon
- Sardines and other small canned fish (in water or brine)
- Ricotta cheese
- Low-fat cottage cheese
- Low-fat paneer
- Greek yogurt
- Egg whites or whole eggs
- Soy/tofu
- Plant-based protein or beans
- Re-Kaged
- KAGED MUSCLE KASEIN
- Micropure Whey Isolate
- Beef
- Skinless poultry
- Pork
- Bison
- Ground meats
- Game meats
- Tilapia
- Tuna

CARBOHYDRATES

The strength and endurance workouts in the MAN of IRON program are highly glycolytic in nature, which means your body will require a specific type of energy in order to perform at its maximum capacity.

To make this diet work for you, you also need to consume plenty of fiber from sources like leafy green vegetables. The gut is where your body breaks down all the food you eat and then absorbs it. This is how you recover, grow, and thrive: through nutrient assimilation. In order to sustain perfect gut health, consume a serving of green vegetables with each meal.

Sources of Carbohydrates:

- Quinoa
- Brown rice
- Whole grains like bulgar or spelt
- Raw or cooked vegetables
- Whole, raw fruit
- High-fiber bread
- Oats
- Muesli
- Potatoes
- Sweet potatoes
- Ezekiel Bread
- Couscous
- Salad greens
- Green vegetables

FATS

Fats are a highly efficient form of calories, and they're essential to hormonal health. You may find your stomach doesn't like it if you eat them around your endurance workouts, so experiment with timing to determine your tolerance.

Sources of Fats:

- Extra-virgin coconut oil
- Olive oil
- Avocados and avocado oil
- Nuts and seeds
- Fish
- Natural nut butters
- Egg Yolks

WATER AND OTHER FLUIDS

It's easy to forget the role water plays in any training program and overall health. Keeping your body hydrated around the clock is absolutely crucial to burning fat, building muscle, aiding recovery, and guaranteeing optimized performance at every workout.

For this MAN of IRON program, you need to consume a minimum of 1 gallon per day, sometimes more, depending on the climate you live in and how much you find you sweat during the endurance training. To further the hydrating properties of your water, I recommend adding Hydra-Charge 3-4 times per day to benefit from the five naturally occurring electrolytes.

During long rides and runs, hydration is the difference between feeling good and feeling like death. Always take more fluid than you need. Camelbaks and other hydration packs are a no-brainer. Don't forget to drink while you're swimming as well—you sweat more than you think in the water.

Fluids:

- Water
- Coconut water
- Black coffee
- Green tea
- Unsweetened and cream-free teas

- Water flavored with Hydra-Charge, Fermented BCAAs, and Fermented Glutamine

NUTRITION ON THE WEEKEND

On any given Saturday, you might be undertaking an 80-mile bike ride through hilly terrain in hot weather. Other times, you may be doing a long bike ride plus a short run, or a long run and an open-water swim, or some other combination of the three triathlon components.

Fueling for this much variety is more art than science. You will have to figure out what works for you through trial and error, but I've included three strategies to help figure out your weekend fueling plan:

Weigh yourself at the start and the end of your activity. The first time you do this after a long endurance workout, you may be surprised by how much weight you've lost. Some of that is from sweat loss, so being proactive about drinking water mixed with Hydra-Charge will help. But you also need to eat enough calories to make up for what you've lost. My goal on weekend training days is to stay within three pounds of where I started the day. I weigh myself once training is done, then alter my future plan accordingly.

Track calorie burn as much as possible. I used a power-tracking stationary watt bike, a Garmin 920XT watch, a heart rate monitor, and a Garmin Connect App to help track progress and calories burned with relative accurately. You may not have access to that type of equipment, but I recommend investing in a heart rate monitor and an app to help calculate calorie burn during your long runs, rides, and swims. Make sure to eat enough to match that burn, and then some.

Start your journey with a shake. When heading out for a long bike ride or run, I found that it was easier to drink a lot of my carbohydrates rather than eating them. Here is my personal blend of a carb and protein shake that help the body stay fueled and stave off muscle loss:

- Bananas, 3
- Dates, 8
- Oats, 1/2 cup
- Honey, 2 tbsp
- Re-Kaged Protein, 2 scoops
- Water, as necessary to blend

During the ride, further fuel yourself with things like dried fruit, protein pancakes, energy balls, and protein powder as needed. For the rest of the day, eat as if it is any normal day of the week unless you need to make up for excess calorie burn.

Yes, this will launch your daily calories through the roof. But you must embrace it fearlessly! This is a whole new world of training, and you'll need to fuel yourself like a high-performance machine to perform like one.

I also use a healthy food preparation and delivery company called Nutrition Solutions here in the USA which delivers high protein pancakes, protein bars, and protein donuts, which were particularly helpful during longer runs and rides through training and through the IRONMAN. I have also found a company called Picky Bars founded by top-seeded IRONMAN athlete Jesse Thomas to be a great, healthy, natural fuel source of bars that are light on the stomach and easy to carry.

My girlfriend, Sunshine, who is a Half-IRONMAN competitor, makes "no-bake" energy balls which are quick and easy to make but extremely efficient to digest for needed output. With the inclusion of Re-Kaged protein, they are a great anti-catabolic bomb to maintain muscle while dominating the miles on the run and bike. The recipe is at the end of this chapter, along with other recipes for breakfast, lunch, and dinner.

Sample Meal Plan for a Day:

MEAL 1
8gg whites, 1 yolk, 1 cup of oats, strawberries, blueberries, pineapple, chia seeds and chopped walnuts.

MEAL 2
Post Weight Training Workout – 1 scoop of Re-Kaged.

MEAL 3
160gm of white fish, 1.5 cup of quinoa, green veggies.

MEAL 4
180gm of Tofu, 1 cup of brown rice and salad.

MEAL 5
150gm of lean red meat, 1.5 cup of sweet potatoes and green veggies.

MEAL 6.
1 Scoop of KAGED MUSCLE KASEIN, chopped pineapple and chopped almonds.

NUTRITION TIPS

- The more advanced your training, the more dialing in your nutrition matters. Yes, you may be craving more junk food (and booze) than ever, but if you're aiming for an elite goal, it has no place in the mix.

- Breakfast burrito, anyone? Just cook up egg whites, tomatoes, fat-free cheese, and mushrooms, and wrap them in a whole-grain tortilla with your sauce of choice.

- If you're traveling and trying to get in quality training, it can be tough to stay on schedule with your meals—and even tougher to stay hydrated. Both are equally important, though. Don't wait until you're gasping during a workout to remember to drink, or your performance will go down in a hurry!

- If you don't have time to eat, drink your meals. A Whey Protein Isolate shake blended with ice, water, oats, fruits, and nuts can make the perfect tasty meal replacement on the go.

RECIPES

Breakfast
WILD RIDE WAFFLES
INGREDIENTS:

- 1 cup buckwheat flour
- 8 egg whites
- 1/4 cup berries
- 1 teaspoon cinnamon
- 1 small lemon
- 1 teaspoon pink salt
- 2 tablespoons crushed walnuts
- 1 scoop Kaged Muscle Supps Vanilla Kasein
- 1/2 cup almond milk

DIRECTIONS:

Put everything except for the lemon in a small bowl and mix well.

Grate the lemon and squeeze the juice out into the bowl. (Watch out for seeds!)

Add almond milk as needed until you get the desired thickness.

Pour batter on waffle iron or griddle and cook until browned on both sides.

Top off with low-fat Greek yogurt and berries.

BISON BREAKFAST BOWL
INGREDIENTS:

5 oz organic ground bison

1/2 cup sweet potatoes, cubed

1 teaspoon cumin

1 teaspoon paprika

1 teaspoon turmeric

1 teaspoon cayenne pepper

(leave this out if you don't like spicy)

1 teaspoon pepper

1 teaspoon pink salt

1/2 cup onion, chopped

1/2 cup red bell pepper, chopped

1/2 cup zucchini, chopped

1/4 cup garlic, minced

1/2 cup rainbow chard, chopped

DIRECTIONS:

Wash and chop potatoes. Prep onions, red pepper, zucchini, chard, and garlic.

In a large skillet over medium high heat, spray some avocado or coconut oil in the skillet then add the potatoes, then season
with cumin, paprika, turmeric, cayenne pepper, salt, and pepper.

Mix until combined, then cover the potatoes and continue to cook for 20-30 minutes, stirring occasionally.

In another skillet prep the bison. Cook until browned.

Remove the lid from the potatoes. Add the red onions, zucchini, peppers, and garlic. Stir until combined and cook for about ten minutes, stirring occasionally.

While the potatoes finish cooking, grab a bowl to put everything in.

Once the potatoes are done, put them in a bowl then top off with the organic ground bison and rainbow chard.

OPTIONAL: For added calories, throw in a couple fried whole eggs.

BERRY CRUNCH HIGH PROTEIN BREAKFAST OATS

INGREDIENTS:
- 1/2 cup oats
- 1 scoop Kaged Muscle Supps Re-Kaged
- 1 teaspoon cinnamon
- 1 teaspoon bee pollen
- 1/2 teaspoon pink salt
- 1/4 cup organic berries
- 1/2 teaspoon chia seeds
- 1/2 teaspoon hemp seeds

DIRECTIONS:
Make your oats and then mix in all the good stuff!

Lunch
VEGAN COBB SALAD

INGREDIENTS:

- 1 cup organic spring mix
- 1 cup butterleaf lettuce
- 1 cup romaine lettuce
- 1/2 cup cooked chickpeas
- 1/2 cup cooked quinoa
- 1/4 cup sliced cherry tomatoes
- 1/4 cup sliced cucumbers
- 1/4 cup zucchini, cut into cubes
- 1/4 cup green beans, cut into small pieces
- 1/4 cup grilled asparagus
- 1/2 cup roasted beets
- 1 teaspoon hemp seeds
- 1 teaspoon sunflower seeds
- 1/2 avocado, sliced

DIRECTIONS:

Throw everything in a bowl and mix it up.
Dress with your favorite dressing.

PB BANANA AND TURKEY BACON TOAST

INGREDIENTS:

- 1 slice of organic sprouted bread
- 1 tablespoon creamy peanut butter
- 1/2 banana, sliced
- 2 strips of turkey bacon

DIRECTIONS:

Toast your bread and then spread peanut butter all over it.
Cook your bacon to your desired crispy level and then add
to toast. Top off with bananas. Now drool.

CHICKEN AND VEG BENTO BOWL

INGREDIENTS:

1 cup cooked brown rice
5 oz grilled chicken
1/2 red bell pepper, sliced
1/4 cup red onion, chopped
1/4 cup broccoli, cut into small pieces
1/4 cup shredded carrots
Handful of cilantro
1 tablespoon liquid aminos sauce
1 small lime, juiced

DIRECTIONS:

Add rice and top with chicken and vegetables. Pour liquid aminos and lime juice over the top and enjoy.

Dinner
STEAK AND SWEET POTATO TACOS

INGREDIENTS:

- 6 oz lean steak
- 1/2 cup cooked sweet potato, cut into small cubes
- 1 red bell pepper, thinly sliced
- 1 onion, thinly sliced
- 1 lime
- 1 tomato, cut into small cubes
- 1 cup organic spring mix
- 3 organic corn tortillas

DIRECTIONS:

Grill steak to desired wellness level. Add spices as desired.

Saute potatoes with bell peppers and onions until the edges begin to crisp. Add spices and salt to taste.

Load up your tortilla with steak, sweet potato mixture, tomatoes, and spring mix. Squeeze some lime over it all and enjoy.

BLACK BEAN ZOODLE BOWL

This meal packs a lot of flavor and is low in carbs. When you're consuming most of your carbs during training, it's good to eat a dinner that is on the lighter side.

You're going to need one big bowl and a good knife and cutting board. Start by putting the zoodles in the bowl and then layering the rest of the vegetables on top in this order: black beans with spinach, roasted delicata squash, red bell pepper, corn, avocado, pepitas, and mango salsa.

INGREDIENTS:

ZOODLES:

2 zucchinis cut into noodles (you'll need a veggie spiraler or you can buy them pre-noodled)

2 tablespoons lemon juice

BLACK BEANS WITH SPINACH:

1 can black beans

2 handfuls of spinach

1/4 cup red onions

1/2 teaspoon olive oil

1/2 teaspoon pink salt

FEGGIE AND NUT MIX:

1/2 red bell pepper, diced into cubes

1/4 cup corn

1/2 avocado, sliced or cubed

1/2 cup grape tomatoes, sliced

1 tbs pepitas, roasted and salted

1 tsp sunflower seeds, roasted and salted

ROASTED DELICATA SQUASH:

1 delicata squash

1 teaspoon cumin

1/2 tablespoon olive oil

MANGO SALSA:

2 ripe mangoes, peeled, pitted, and diced (about 3 cups)

1 small red onion, peeled and diced

1-2 jalapenos, seeded and diced

1/2 cup chopped fresh cilantro, loosely packed

juice of one lime

DIRECTIONS:

Mix zoodles in with lemon juice to taste and add to bowl.

Cook onion in olive oil over medium heat until soft. Add the can of beans and sprinkle with pink salt. Stir and let it cook for a minute, then add spinach. Continue cooking until spinach has wilted and is incorporated into the beans.

Cut, slice, and roast everything and add to zoodle bowl.

Preheat oven to 400 degrees.

Prepare the squash by cutting it in half lengthwise. Use a tablespoon to scoop out the seeds. Slice squash into 1/4 inch-thick half moons.

Place squash on a baking pan covered with aluminum foil. Toss with olive oil and sprinkle with cumin.

Cook for approximately 20 minutes. The goal is for the squash to be soft, but slightly caramelized on the bottom. Once done, grab a few pieces and add them to your zoodle bowl.

Toss all ingredients together until combined. Season with salt and pepper if needed. Top off zoodle bowl.

TURKEY LETTUCE WRAPS

INGREDIENTS:

FILLING
1 pound lean ground turkey
2 tablespoons garlic salt
1/4 cup onion, minced
1/4 cup red bell pepper, minced
1/4 cup zucchini, minced
1/2 cup cooked rice (optional)

PEANUT SAUCE
1 tablespoon peanut butter
1 tablespoon fresh lemon or lime juice
1 tablespoon olive oil
1 tablespoon apple cider vinegar
1/2 teaspoon cayenne pepper

WRAPS
1 large head of organic butter leaf lettuce,
leaves washed and pulled apart

DIRECTIONS:

To make the filling, cook the turkey on medium high heat in a saute pan. Once the turkey turns brown, add in the onion, red bell pepper, zucchini, and garlic salt. Cover and let cook for another 10 minutes, stirring every now and again.

To make the sauce, combine the peanut butter, lemon or lime juice, olive oil, and vinegar in a small bowl. Mix everything together and adjust ingredients to achieve pourable consistency.

Let filling cool for a bit and then scoop into lettuce leaves and top with peanut sauce. Roll up or fold over and eat the wrap with your hands.

Snacks
SUNSHINE'S ENERGY BALLS

INGREDIENTS:

- 1/2 cup oats
- 1 cup pitted medjool dates
- 1/2 cup almonds
- 1 teaspoon cinnamon
- 1/2 teaspoon turmeric
- 1/4 teaspoon ginger
- 1/2 teaspoon cacao
- 1 teaspoon pink salt
- 1 scoop Kaged Muscle Supplements Re-Kaged

DIRECTIONS:

Combine everything in food processor.

Blend until pieces start sticking together.

Roll into little balls.

PROTEIN RICE CAKES

INGREDIENTS:

- 4 organic brown rice cakes
- 1 scoop Kaged Muscle Supplements Vanilla (or Chocolate) Kasein
- 1 teaspoon bee pollen
- Handful of blueberries
- 1/2 cup filtered water

DIRECTIONS:

Mix the Kasein in with a little bit of water until you reach a creamy consistency.

Spread Kasein on the rice cakes.

Top off with bee pollen and blueberries.

TURKEY BACON AND EGGS RICE CAKE

INGREDIENTS:

2 cups uncooked calrose or other medium grain "sticky" rice
3 cups water
8 strips of turkey bacon
3 eggs
2 tablespoons liquid amino acids
1 teaspoon salt

DIRECTIONS:

Combine water and rice in rice cooker.

While rice is cooking, chop up turkey bacon into small pieces and fry in a saute pan. When crispy, soak up extra fat with paper towels.

Beat eggs in small bowl and then scramble in saute pan.

In a large bowl, combine the cooked rice, turkey bacon, and scrambled eggs. Add liquid aminos to taste. After mixing, press into a 8-inch square baking pan.

Top with salt.

Cut and wrap individual cakes.

CHAPTER 8
SUPPLEMENTS

Anyone out there who says supplements don't do anything is un-educated. The levels of vitamins and minerals in our food are not as high as they used to be. With the intensity level of this program, you are not going to adequately recover without supplements. You can sleep 16 hours per day if you want, but you won't produce the nutrients your body needs. Mentally, you can push through a work-out without your body utilizing the correct balance, but you can't do that for too many days in a row. Your tank will run out of gas and you won't be able to perform.

Being heavily involved at the top of the bodybuilding food chain for almost 20 years, I've taken a lot of supplements and lab tested a lot of supplements. Unfortunately, as I discovered, many of the well-known brands came up substantially short of the ingredients they supposedly contained. Not only that, heavy metal contaminants, banned substances, untested and generic ingredients and pro-tein spiking became more apparent the more testing procedures I encountered. In 2013, I decided explore the possibility of creating my own line with very best formulators and manufactures in the world, who I also happen to know. After 18 months of testing, we

"

**WITH THE INTENSITY
LEVEL OF THIS
PROGRAM, YOU
ARE NOT GOING
TO ADEQUATELY
RECOVER WITHOUT
SUPPLEMENTS.**

"

decided to launch a line that had fermented, organic, patented, and 3rd party tested ingredients that were naturally flavored and adherent to heavy metal contaminant tests, certified free of banned substances, and that could merge the health sector with the performance sector. In 2014 we launched KAGED MUSCLE. I am fully aware that I may come across as a salesman here, but I encourage you to look at the ratings and reviews online to remove any bias. I am only educating you on this quality brand because I believe it to be the best in the word (we have won multiple awards from Bodybuilding.com and Vitamin Shoppe) and I only wish someone had educated me as I try to educate others on the importance of quality ingredients over promotional marketing.

For my MAN of IRON training, I created a custom supplement stack to help get the most out of my combination of hybrid weights workouts and endurance training. As with the nutrition plan in the previous chapter, work to master your airtight system during the week, and then use what you've learned to tackle the unpredictable nature of weekend workouts.

The nice thing about long rides and runs is that you need water during them anyway, so adding a scoop of crucial supplemental nutrients to a bottle you're already carrying doesn't add any weight. If you bike or run with a small satchel, pocketed jersey, or other garb that allows you to carry small items, predose your supplements in small baggies and keep them packed away.

I've included descriptions of the main supplements I used in this program below:

PRE-KAGED

Pre-Kaged pre-workout powder boosts your energy, strength, and endurance so you can train harder and sustain high intensity levels.* It's the perfect blend of premium grade ingredients to prime your central nervous system, increase nitric oxide, and give your muscles the edge they need to perform maximally.*

The Pre-Kaged formula packs 6.5g of PURE L-Citrulline giving you enhanced muscle pumps each and every time you train.*

Each serving contains 3.5 grams of rapidly dissolving, instantized BCAAs for easy mixing. The BCAA blend of leucine, isoleucine, and valine uses a proven 2:1:1 ratio and is readily absorbed into your system where it goes directly to muscles, delivering fast support for protein synthesis.* The addition of 3 grams of leucine further fuels protein synthesis, allowing you to maximize muscle gains.*

To add more fuel to the fire: There are 1.5 grams of highly absorbable, concentrated Creatine HCL in every serving. What's more, the patented ingredients CarnoSyn (beta-alanine) and Beta-Power (betaine) are designed to work together with Creatine HCl to fend off fatigue.*

A neuro support matrix packed with taurine, L-tyrosine, and PurCaf organic caffeine work to promote heightened mental clarity and focus.*

Other than taking this before my weights workouts, I generally will use this in a race capacity of a 70.3 or full IRONMAN during the ride section of the 3 disciplines for the final boost.

IN-KAGED

In-Kaged is designed to push your body harder for longer in the gym by boosting your energy, strength, and endurance levels.*

Each serving of In-Kaged packs in 1.6g of CarnoSyn beta-alanine, one of the purest forms of beta-alanine available. This patented ingredient has been scientifically formulated to boost muscle carnosine levels, enabling you to blast through rep after rep without fatigue.*

In-Kaged also includes 5g of rapidly dissolving, instantized fermented BCAAs so your muscles can soak them up faster and kickstart protein synthesis.* A combination of taurine, L-tyrosine, and PurCaf organic caffeine provides neuro support, heightening mental clarity and laser-like focus as you train.*

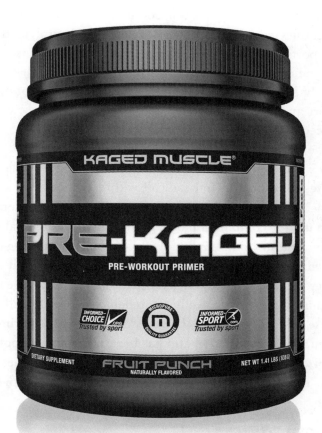

Similar to my intake of Pre-Kaged, I generally will use this during weights workouts, in a race capacity of a 70.3 or full IRONMAN, and during the run section of the 3 disciplines for the final boost.

HYDRA-CHARGE

Hydra-Charge is a hydrating formula that provides you with calcium, phosphorous, magnesium, sodium, and potassium to ensure you get the vital micronutrients you need for electrolyte function.* It supports hydration and the body's natural defenses before, during, and after intense training.* Hydra-Charge has five essential electrolytes from freeze-dried coconut water for superior hydration support and is combined with SPECTRA, which is scientifically balanced to support antioxidant potential.*

The SPECTRA high oxygen radical absorbance capacity (ORAC) antioxidant fusion works to boost your body's natural defenses by combating free radicals within the body.*

Each serving of Hydra-Charge electrolyte drink powder is made from a unique combination of vegetable, fruit, and herbal extracts and concentrates, and is naturally flavored for an amazing taste.

Hydra-Charge also contains 1 gram of taurine, a mind-enhancing ingredient that helps you get focused and in the zone each time you train.* Taurine is a well-researched regulator of cell volume because it regulates fluid balance.* As a result, taurine helps maximize muscle function and has been noted to be a potent cell volumizer.* This means not only will your muscle bellies appear bigger, they'll also be provided an indirect stimulus for muscle growth.*

RE-KAGED

Want to know the real secret to building muscle, getting stronger and improving endurance every day? RECOVERY. When you push your body to its limits, you're creating micro tears. To build that body and the split times, those tears need to be repaired. Even if

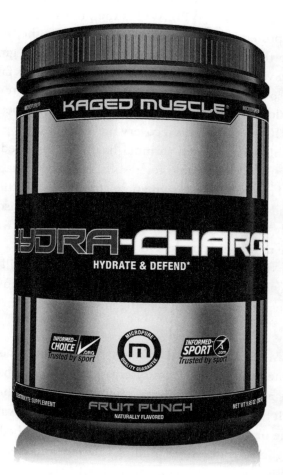

you're following a sound diet and getting plenty of rest, your body needs a little help to see results faster. That's where Re-Kaged steps in.

Re-Kaged post workout protein is designed to help you build muscle and recover at light speed.* Each serving packs 28 grams of Whey Protein Isolate (WPI). WPI is the purest and fastest digesting of all proteins, releasing its amino acids into the bloodstream quickly so they can get to work stimulating muscle growth.* Replenishing your muscles with amino acids also means faster recovery times so you can get back to the gym and crush your workouts.* The addition of fermented glutamine, BetaPower (betaine), and Creatine HCl complete this recovery fuel complex.*

The third-party tested formula has been reviewed endlessly and meticulously calibrated for results. It's been enhanced using patented ProHydrolayse enzymatic technology and full spectrum amino acids to maximize protein absorption and muscle repair.* Put simply, it helps your body absorb more protein while at the same time minimizing muscle soreness.

Other than taking this post weights workout, I will drink this during my longer riding sessions along with carbs coming from fruits for extra energy while keeping me anti-catabolic.

C-HCl

KAGED MUSCLE patented Creatine HCl powder is a highly concentrated, ultra-pure form of creatine proven to have greater solubility and predicted bioavailability than any other form of creatine. It has been shown to completely dissolve in water, leaving no residue or sediment behind—meaning it's absorbed instead of left sitting in your intestines, pulling in water, and creating gastrointestinal issues commonly associated with creatine. That means less bloating, diarrhea, gas, and cramping. Because of creatine HCL's increased absorption and predicted bioavailability, athletes report they can reap all the benefits of creatine monohydrate

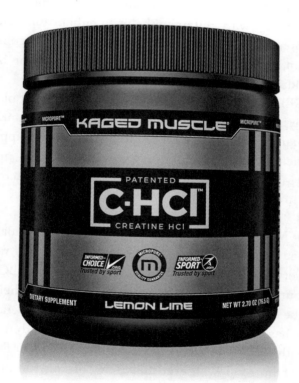

supplementation with lower amounts of creatine HCL. You're also able to skip the loading phase normally required with non-synthesized creatine.

GLUTAMINE POWDER

Glutamine is the most abundant amino acid in the human body, important to several processes including muscle growth. When your body is depleted of glutamine, such as after an intense workout, it cannot build muscle and may become over trained. Supplementing with glutamine helps to enhance muscle growth, reduce muscle breakdown especially in those undergoing calorie restriction, and support recovery.* Glutamine also combats lactic acid buildup that leads to fatigue.*

KAGED MUSCLE Glutamine is fermented from plant-based raw materials, not made from bird feathers or human hair like most on the market (yes, it's true!). This premium-quality supplement is vegan-friendly, and is free of heavy metals, impurities, and toxins. KAGED MUSCLE Glutamine is also kosher and gluten free.

BCAA 2:1:1

KAGED MUSCLE BCAA powder has been formulated from fermented BCAAs, blended together in a proven 2:1:1 ratio. Each 5-gram serving features rapidly dissolving, instantized BCAAs. The faster your muscles soak up these amino acids, you'll help to stave off fatigue and soreness, and speed recovery.* The science-backed formula has also been perfected to help your body feel better, faster, with clean ingredients free of artificial colors or flavors.* It's perfect for those following even the strictest of diets, formulated with vegetable sourced, vegan-friendly fermented BCAAs.

Your body needs the highest quality fuel to ensure proper recovery so you can crush every workout. That's what sets KAGED MUSCLE BCAA 2:1:1 formula apart. Our premium grade

BCAAs stimulate protein synthesis to help rebuild your muscles,* even more so than just protein on its own. This means that you'll repair and rebuild muscle tissue at a faster rate.*

These statements have not been evaluated by the Food and Drug Administration. This product is not intended to diagnose, treat, cure, or prevent any disease.

Below is a schedule of my supplement intake during the training process.

WEIGHT-TRAINING OR HYBRID TRAINING DAYS
Pre-Kaged- 30 minutes pre-workout
In-Kaged- during workout
Re-Kaged- 1 serving post-workout but pre-cardio

DURING POST-WORKOUT HOUR, AFTER CARDIO
Hydra-Charge- 3 serving
BCAA 2:1:1 Powder- 3 serving
Glutamine Powder- 4 serving
C-HCl- 2 serving

NON-TRAINING DAYS
Hydra-Charge- 3 serving
BCAA 2:1:1 Powder- 3 serving
Glutamine Powder- 4 serving
C-HCl- 2 serving

LONG CARDIO SESSIONS, FIRST 2 HOURS
(1ST WATER BOTTLE)
Hydra-Charge- 3 serving
BCAA 2:1:1 Powder- 3 serving
Glutamine Powder- 4 serving
C-HCl- 2 serving

LONG CARDIO SESSIONS, FIRST 2 HOURS
(2ND WATER BOTTLE)
Re-Kaged- 1 serving

LONG CARDIO SESSIONS, SECOND 2+ HOURS
(3RD WATER BOTTLE)
In-Kaged- 1 serving

LONG CARDIO SESSIONS, SECOND 2+ HOURS
(4TH WATER BOTTLE)
Re-Kaged- 1 serving

SUPPLEMENT TIPS

- The timing of your food and supplemens matters for muscle growth.

- The more active we are, the more we oxidize and utilize nutrients such as amino acids, so we need to eat more and supplement to compensate.

- Soil is undernourished due to over-harvesting—thus, so is the food that we eat today. Supplementation is needed to compensate for lack of nutrients in food and to enhance performance.

CHAPTER 9
MENTALITY

One aspect of training and competition that people sometimes overlook takes place not in the body, but in the mind. Competing against myself isn't going to come from my genetic potential, athletic ability, or talent. It's going to come from what's going on from the neck up. I could have things holding me back from the neck down—injuries, sore muscles, fatigue—but I know everything from the neck up—my brain, application, discipline, passion, motivation—is what will make the difference.

Do what you fear—don't fear what you do. At one point in training, I needed to fit in a long bike ride but I'd just returned from a long flight and knew I had a crazy week ahead of me. I thought, *It would be nice just to have the afternoon or evening off.* Doubts and excuses and complacency attacked me, but I fought against them and told myself, *No, no no, I've committed to this. My word is absolutely everything. All I've got to do is go through the motion and get out there and I will evolve. I will get better; I'll be closer to succeeding.* Once I went out on the bike, I ended up riding farther than I planned. I was having a difficult time finding motivation within myself, so I listened to the audiobook "Extreme Ownership" and it helped me push myself to the next level, past where Kris Gethin normally would have stopped. If my own voice is overriding positive thoughts and I don't have a coach or a training partner, then sometimes I need an external motivating voice to push me along. These voices can come from music, podcasts, looking at a poster of an athlete...if you need inspiration, go out and look for it.

BRETT SUTTON'S COACHING METHOD

Brett Sutton is a top triathlete coach in Switzerland, but his methods are regarded as controversial. He's trained athletes such as Chrissie Wellington and Siri Lindey into world champions. Of course, they had practiced visualization and visualized winning, but Sutton completely broke them mentally down.

When Siri arrived, her luggage was delayed and he told her, "You're getting on the turbo trainer."

She replied, "Well, my luggage hasn't shown up."

"Then you're going to wear what you're wearing," he responded. Siri looked down and she was in jeans. She ended up wearing them as she rode the turbo trainer for three hours. The following day, early in the morning before breakfast, they went out on a long, hilly cycle ride. At the end Sutton took her down to the bottom of the mountain and said, "Alright, now walk 20 kilometers back up the mountain to your lodging." Siri learned to just focus on surviving each day of training, and lost sight of her vision and dream to become a world champion.

Because she stopped dreaming, she started applying and putting in all the brickwork needed to lead that road to a journey of success—ultimate success. I think that's what a lot of people miss today. I have a friend who tried to compete in an IRONMAN just recently, but he didn't even get out of the swim on time because he didn't have respect for the journey. All he thought about was the event, and he told everybody he was competing, but he didn't respect the training—what was directly in front of him.

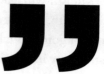

CONSISTENCY WITH DISCIPLINE CONTAINS MONOTONY.

EMBRACE REALITY AND CONSISTENCY

Most people look at the world how they want it to be, not how it really is. As soon as you become real with the pain and adversity that you may have to overcome and respect that, then the chances of you succeeding are much higher. There are a lot of people out on that IRONMAN track who are dealing with as much pain as you, if not more, but they're going to finish ahead of you because they've respected the journey. They've become conditioned to the pain; they know that it's only temporary and it's something they must respect and even embrace.

I always measure things by very, very short-term goals. If I'm getting ready for a bodybuilding show, I don't think about the 12 weeks ahead of me; I think about my next meal—am I going to get my next meal in on time?—because I need to be prepared. I haven't missed a meal in over 18 years now, because I'm always thinking about making sure I get the next one. It doesn't matter if I'm traveling; doesn't matter if I get invited to a social gathering. That is my goal because I know it will lead to my ultimate success and I want to take care of my health. I want to make sure I'm not having blood sugar crashes; I'm not going to have erratic cravings; I want to make sure that I don't strain my internal organs by taking in massive meals. I want very small, easy-to-digest meals. I know if I have a smaller meal, it's not going to sap as much energy from me and I'm going to get more stuff done.

This mentality carries over into the gym. You look at the set and the exercise in front of you—a lot of people would say, *I've got three sets yet, so I'll save myself for the last one.* During a bike ride I might think to myself, *Should I finish early? By the time I get home it will be 8:30 p.m. and I need to get up at 4 a.m. tomorrow morning to film in the gym then hit a swim...maybe I'll be a bit too fatigued.* But I stop talking to myself like that and think, *No. You worry about tomorrow, tomorrow. You will adapt.* Don't think of the training program as a six-month process—approach it day by day. You think about what you must do today, which will lead to tomorrow. You can go to bed tonight, cross it off, and go, *Okay, I was a success today, let's start again tomorrow, instead of saving that room for the possibility that I can make this up.* You can't make it up. You can't really get ahead either, but you can stay on track.

Focus your motivation on consistency. It's not going to be your equipment; it's not going to be how fit you are; it's not going to be your genetic potential; it's not going to be the injury that holds you back. It's consistency that will build you up every single day. But that consistency must be broken into very short, manageable goals, and if that means writing it down, having an alert on your phone, creating a sense of urgency—that is going to be the main thing that's going to get you from Point A to Point B. Control your environment, don't let it control you.

REWIRE YOUR BRAIN

I keep an app on my phone that's a countdown of how many years I have left on this earth. It counts down how many meals I have left. I've put in there that, on average, I believe I'm going to live to 100 years old—anything further from that is going to be a bonus, great, fantastic—but at the moment, I'm nearing the halfway point to 100 years. So, I have a sense of urgency to make every day count. I don't want to be stuck in traffic. I don't want to have mindless conversations. I don't want to be stuck in conference calls unless it's going to have some sort of benefit, because for me, wasting time is going to be worse than spending or blowing money or giving it away. People would never give all their money away—well, some people do. If I'm out on the bike, if I'm in the gym, I want to make sure that the time I spend there is very, very efficient. Because I have a sense of urgency just like my app is telling me every day. It doesn't make me paranoid. I don't think it's morbid. But I think it's a good sense of urgency to make you accountable to your goals.

This mentality takes some rewiring for sure, much like I rewired myself from training 45 minutes with extreme intensity to training for the long haul of an IRONMAN. It took me a several months to rewire my brain to think like that. You're going to have to work at rewiring your circuitry a little bit, because just like it takes time to pick up bad habits, now it's going to take time to remove those bad habits, and then it's going to take even more time to pick up the new habits. You replace the components in your circuit board and that becomes the norm. To me, waking up at four o'clock in the morning is the norm. It's not for many people—it's definitely not for my girlfriend—but for her to be up at midnight is the norm. I can't do that.

We recently spent a weekend in Las Vegas for work. At 9 p.m., I was ready to return to the hotel and go to bed, but society pressure says in Las Vegas the night is a time to go out and party. Well, can you think how many other decisions your brain must process like that? Oh, we should do this because it's a social norm. It's the weekend, so it's a social norm. We switch off on the weekends because we're not supposed to work. There are so many decisions influenced by your environment or by people around you, and you really have to find yourself to navigate your desired path. I had to get up early in the morning to catch my flight then go on a long bike ride. I couldn't go out and party, then be successful in my true priorities.

You must really look at yourself and your brain's thought process from an outside perspective instead of accepting the internal habits it has created. We face 3,500 decisions every day—but think, how many of those decisions are possibly wrong or confusing, and you actually go for them? Maybe it's because of your upbringing. What sort of habits have I picked up from my parents? Are they good? Are they bad? Does it matter? As long as I'm acknowledging it, and I'm aware of it, then I can make better decisions. Don't make decisions through emotion. When I didn't want to go train on the bike, that was based on emotion. I sometimes had

CONTROL YOUR ENVIRONMENT, DON'T LET IT CONTROL YOU.

to be practical and write it down, going: Okay, what are the pros and cons of me staying at home right now just doing nothing, or going out and getting this ride done? When you write those pros and cons out, emotion is taken out of the equation. I went for that ride. Hybrid training is demanding, and you'll have to suffer for your art. For some people, discipline is normal. It's just robotic after a while. But for some others, it's not. It's a struggle. It's a definite struggle. Change your perception on what life really is out there, and how we can grasp it.

MAINTAIN INSPIRATION

At the doctor's office I go to for cryotherapy, there's a woman who also comes in for treatment who used to be a professional triathlete. Two weeks before she was going to compete in Kona, she was knocked down by a car in the desert, and now she's paralyzed from the waist down. She's very determined to get the feeling back in her feet. She's in the office three days a week, working with Dr. Jason Watson. She does so much stuff at home as well—she'll spend anywhere between five and seven hours a day working on herself, absolutely convinced that she'll get the feeling back in her legs. The doctors don't think she will. But Dr. Watson is positive that she can improve. Her situation made me think, *Wow, we really need to grasp everything we possibly can, because who knows what's around the corner?* I should be motivated; I should want to influence others. People learn by observation. We are a crowd source of inspiration. I can't do this by myself, but if I inspire someone to do a triathlon, then maybe someone else will do a marathon. Maybe someone else within that family who watched that person getting ready for a marathon is going to actually start eating better and taking better care of themselves. When you actually start putting your journey out there and potentially start inspiring other people, it motivates you a little bit more. You're accountable to yourself then, because

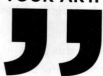

**HYBRID TRAINING IS
DEMANDING, AND
YOU'LL HAVE TO
SUFFER FOR YOUR ART.**

you're putting your sincerity on the line if you don't go out there and do it, if you don't eat the food necessary to fuel yourself, to allow you to recover.

ATHLETE INSPIRATION

A hybrid athlete who inspires me is Ross Edgely. Ross looks like he could win a bodybuilding show at any time during the year. The guy is huge, muscular, and stays in great shape. Not only that, he completes feats of unique unimaginable endurance and strength. He once completed a 70.3 distance triathlon while carrying and towing a 45-kilogram tree to raise awareness of climate change. He has also rope climbed the equivalent height of Mount Everest, and created the "World's Strongest Marathon" by towing a 1,400-kilogram Mini Countryman car 26.2 miles.

His unique use and versatility of muscle is extremely inspiring. Not only that, he always uses these feats to help others in need, create awareness for the world, and encourage muscular health and fitness in our industry. The world of Hybrid Athleticism will grow fast with Ross Edgely on the forefront. You can find inspiration from a variety of sources.

Many people in this day and age want the results. They want the job promotion, to own the business, the nice car, to get first place, but they're not willing to put in the hard work. Consistency with discipline contains monotony, and that's what it all comes down to at the end of the day. Many people dream and visualize, which is good for the short term. But if they visualize winning a certain event, and it stays nothing more than a dream, they won't address the hard task that is directly in front of them to achieve it.

Another hybrid athlete who inspires me is named Ben Greenfield. Ben served as president of the triathlon club for his university while maintaining a physique of 215 pounds and 3 percent body fat.

He then went on to compete in 12 IRONMAN triathlons, win top bowhunting competitions, and complete the Spartan delta—the Spartan Sprint, Spartan Super, and Spartan Beast races, all in a calendar year. And these are just a few of his notable accomplishments! As a hybrid athlete, Ben illustrates what it looks like when one sheds societal norms and expectations to pursue one's full potential.

We're hunters, we're gatherers, but when everything is done for us, we become purposeless. What am I here for? Especially with competitive athletes, when they retire, many fall into depression or alcoholism because they've lost their way. They question why they're on this earth, what their new role is. It can take them several years, if they do find their way, to find out who they really are—and it's all based on the journey. It's not the competitive first place against the other person who came first or second or whatever, because it's all about improvement. We can't all be the best bodybuilders; we can't all be the best triathletes. But we can become better, and that's what we should be striving for: making better decisions, becoming fitter, becoming healthier, getting full residency of our lives because a lot of people don't. You look at a lot of people who don't have residence of themselves, really not just physically but mentally, too. They search for motivation like it's an external force and then they can't seem to stop themselves from eating self-destructing foods. And if they were just to learn to rewire themselves a little bit and become more motivated through the influences I've just mentioned—and it may start with something very, very small—then they're going to be much happier. If you're happier, you're going to be a little bit more confident, you're going to have a little bit more energy, you're going to become a little bit more active. And that motivation just comes full circle, then.

But—as I've said before—acknowledge what you actually have and don't take anything for granted—don't focus on the position, focus on being a better version of yourself. If I get a good time in the IRONMAN, or even just finish it, that's my first place; that's a success to me because I've been able to do that, I've promised people I'll do it, I've given myself my word—my word is everything. Once I succeed, great. Will it be my goal next week? Next year? I don't know. Who knows? But if I accomplish something else, if I become a vegan, if I run an ultramarathon, then that's something. It's all about crossing off the notches so I can look at the app on my phone and go, *Yeah, I did something with myself*. I was able to apply and evolve.

"ACKNOWLEDGE WHAT YOU ACTUALLY HAVE AND DON'T TAKE ANYTHING FOR GRANTED—DON'T FOCUS ON THE POSITION, FOCUS ON BEING A BETTER VERSION OF YOURSELF."

MENTALITY TIPS

- Failure is part of the fun. What's the point of doing something if it's easy?

- Some days will be harder than others, but it's days like this that really count. Because anybody can get through the bloody easy times, can't they? Successful people in all ways, all manners, all shapes and forms, sometimes do shit they don't want to do.

- Distance running, biking, swimming—they're all quite tranquil once you find your rhythm. Or, at least, they can be. Try to find peace where you can.

- Feeling sluggish? Get to the gym, get the blood flowing to your brain, improve your focus and energy. Then you're going to be able to attack the day, not let it slip away.

- Your runs and rides can't all be adventures, but neither should they all be treadmill or stationary slogs. Find loops around your home or gym, because there's no substitute for running out in the world.

- Equipment malfunctions happen. And when they do, they ruin training sessions. If you let them, they'll ruin days, as well. Prepare yourself emotionally for some hard moments.

SECTION THREE
RACING

CHAPTER 10
HALF IRONMAN

On June 25th, I competed in the IRONMAN 70.3 in Coeur d'Alene, Idaho. The race took place three months into the training process, so I thought it would be a good marker of my progress and give me an idea of what to expect for the full IRONMAN in August. To give you the same insights as you prepare to race, I've shared the details of my experience below.

THE PREPARATION

The race was on a Sunday, so I traveled to Coeur d'Alene on Thursday to prepare. I don't get nervous as long as I'm not rushed. Friday, I put on my wetsuit and went for an easy 25-minute swim. Its purpose was not to build fitness, but to familiarize myself with the terrain, get the feel of the water, and recover in preparation for the race. In my hotel room I laid out everything I would need for the different transition areas—the visor, sunscreen, sunglasses, shoes with socks inside, and all of my nutrition in shaker bottles without water added yet. Then I went to the athlete check-in and briefing where I picked up my numbers and listened to the rules of the competition.

On Saturday, there was another athlete briefing where the professionals did a question-and-answer session. It was good to listen to them and hear their advice; I'd learned a lot through research, but it was nice to have my findings affirmed. The female pro, Lindsay Corbin, had some good advice, suggesting simply to be present, enjoy the process, and smile every now and again. You're in a beautiful part of the world. Enjoy it. Don't just sweat it out, suffer, and drag yourself over the finish line.

Afterwards I went out for a 30-minute ride on the bike and a 10-minute run. Again, just to loosen things up and make sure everything felt okay and the bike was in good working order. I did one last check in with the bike pressure, put the bike and pump into transition, then went home and went to bed. I went to bed early—about 7:30 p.m.—because I woke up at 3 a.m. to eat.

I ate a big meal consisting of oats with almond butter, some nuts and seeds, and Re-Kaged, my protein powder. Basically about 1,000 calories—a big, big meal—because I knew I would go through those calories, but I didn't want to eat too close to the race. I made my way down to the race at about 4:00. We put the rest of the stuff into the transition, such as the trainers, bike shoes, sunglasses, helmet, and laid everything out.

I went down to the water and got in about 25 minutes before the start, again, just to get used to it. I didn't want to go into the water and have any kind of anxiety from the temperature difference or anything like that. It was all new to me. To see over 2,600 people, all dressed in wetsuits, with all either green caps or pink caps, just waiting to get into the water, was quite a sight. I was surprised at the size of the crowd there at 6 a.m.

THE SWIM

The race began with a rolling start, so I decided to put myself in the category that would take 40-55 minutes. My girlfriend went into that category as well. She wanted to wait until the last category because she didn't feel as confident—not that I'm a strong swimmer by any means—but I felt it would probably be better for her to start a little early. If people passed her, it would be better than having to deal with trying to pass people. The rolling start helped spread everything out. Everything felt surprisingly good. I felt calm. I felt relaxed. There was a little bit of physical contact but it didn't bother me at all. On some occasions people actually came up behind me and I could feel them putting a hand on my hamstring or back, so I slightly increased my tempo and kicked harder at those points. I didn't want to exert too much energy or hurt anybody, but I didn't want to lose any time or have people swimming on top of me.

I made sure that I continued to keep sighting; I was swimming in a much straighter line than I was used to, but I still drifted from side to side between the buoys. It wasn't a perfect line, but I knew I was going in the right direction.

I didn't want to start too fast and run out of gas, so I paced myself, and at the halfway point, I felt good. I knew that I could increase the speed a little bit without overexerting myself for the bike or run. It was a little bit more difficult coming back toward the finish of the swim, because the sun was shining directly toward us. Even though I wore polarized goggles, it was very difficult for me to see so I relied on the people in front as my guide to go in the right direction. One of the things that was quite surprising, because I had some concerns, was that I felt like I had company. It may sound cheesy, but I felt like I had the company of all the viewers of the video series with me. That helped me with the accountability. I thought, *I'm doing a positive thing here. This is much bigger than me. This is possibly opening the opportunity for others who have been on the fence up until now.* Because I knew that gateway was already slowly opening, and an event like the 70.3 was opening it even more. That thought encouraged me and reminded me of the Unique Home for Girls Orphanage I was competing for. The charity was good, that was accountability, but the strongest force to keep me pushing at a decent pace and enjoy the process was knowing that I was bringing viewers and readers along with me.

When I got toward the end of the swim—maybe 5-10 minutes before the finish—I started to visualize everything in regards to the transition. First, I would remove the earplugs, because I'd noticed during previous swims that when I'd come out of the water, my equilibrium would be off and I'd lose balance. Then the goggles, then the cap. I was visualizing stripping the upper half of the wetsuit off, even though I knew there were wetsuit strippers there.

I got out of the water feeling little bit more out of breath than I'd anticipated. I guess because I'd been breathing in a repetitive fashion in the water it felt normal after a while. But I stripped off fine, laid on the floor, allowed the wetsuit strippers who were working in pairs to rip my wetsuit off.

THE BIKE

When I arrived at the transition area I found my bike easily, because when I'd put the bike in the transition amongst a couple thousand other bikes, I saw a tree that had a yellow and blue ribbon around it to use as my center point. That was my marker. I knew my bike was somewhere in that row, and I just had to find the number. When I put everything on—my helmet, my glasses, my belt—I looked back, because the transition went so smoothly I was sure I'd forgotten something. I thought, *Okay, that was smooth, that was easy, let's go.*

I ran out the transition nice and easy. I had my shoes already fixed into the bike, so all I did was put my feet on top of the shoes and started pedaling. When I got out onto the main road, as I started free-wheeling, that's when I put my feet into the shoes again, just to save a little bit of time.

Then we had 54 miles of riding ahead of us, but what was nice about the ride—and this goes for everything—was that it went a lot faster than I figured it would. I suppose when you're out training, you're just there by yourself with your thoughts, and chances are, it's a route that you've already done quite a few times, so time goes a lot slower. But when I was out on the race course with other people, time flew by. People were so encouraging. Even if you passed someone, they told you what a great job you were doing. How awesome. It was an incredibly positive atmosphere. And it was beautiful; a lot of the ride was by the lake. It relaxed me a bit; it chilled me out. I didn't feel nervous at all. I just kept my pace instead of allowing my brain to wander. I kept physically checking myself, asking, *Am I making sure I'm getting the full rotation? Am I relaxed? Am I keeping my upper body still?*

As expected, I was passed a lot on the hills. Every hill we came to, I knew that if there was anybody I'd just passed on the flat or on the decline, chances are they were about to pass me again on the hill. It happened again and again. There were some people competing who I overtook and was overtaken by for the entire ride. Same three or four people. I felt that I used my weight power without overexerting myself on the downhills and flats to go past a lot of people. But then on the uphill, I really had to hold back based on the amount of food that I was eating and fluid I was drinking on the bike. It was a very hilly course. They say it's one of the hardest in the world. It's in the red if you look at the international scale of these events, probably because of the number of hills. I was absolutely fine with the amount of people passing me.

During this time I was making sure—obviously I couldn't do it on the swim—I was taking a drink every 6 minutes, and eating something every 12 minutes. I knew I had to get in around 400 to 500 calories per hour. When I listened to the pros at the athlete briefing, they suggested 100 to 200 calories. They can do that and survive, but I can't do that. So I packed some energy bars made up of dates, oats, cinnamon, turmeric, ginger, manuka honey, bananas, and a scoop of protein powder, and some seeds and nuts. In the pockets on my bike I also packed no-bake energy balls my girlfriend had made in the food processor, along with some carbohydrates. In my drinks bottles I had supplements like glutamine, branched-chain amino acids, Hydra-Charge, and Re-Kaged, which is my protein powder, in a 24-ounce shaker bottle. I also consumed Nutrition Solutions protein pancakes, protein doughnuts, and Pickey Bars. I alternated between the foods—sticking to mostly solid foods—and the drink. I didn't bother stopping at any aid stations—they gave out fluids and all that stuff—but I had everything I needed on my bike.

On the bike I was surprised how sore my butt became because I'd done that mileage before, but maybe as a rookie mistake, I was wearing shorts I hadn't trained in. I'd been waiting for some prints of my KAGED MUSCLE supplement line and Tri-Town to be print-ed on the shorts. It took longer than anticipated, so I hadn't ridden with them.

I quite enjoyed the ride. I passed more people than people passed me, and made up a lot of ground. I obviously had not had as strong a swim as these people, but I felt that I had a little bit of advantage cycling.

It didn't feel like I was lagging at all, timewise. I didn't time my swim, but I wanted to time my ride and my run to ensure I finished before the eight-and-a-half-hour cutoff. I knew I was ahead and I was happy with that. I felt like I'd paced fine and I didn't feel like I'd overexerted myself. We went through town to go back to the transi-tion, which was fantastic because it felt like the whole community of Coeur d'Alene was in the streets, encouraging and shouting at riders, and there were a lot of people out on the freeway with horns, and the volunteers there were awesome and very encouraging. The uplifting feedback made a big difference. The only problem that developed was the heat. Toward the last quarter of the ride it really, really started to get hot.

THE RUN

As I dismounted the bike I felt good. I felt strong. I ran past the people walking the transition, put the bike on the rack, got rid of the helmet, put my training shoes on, which had quick laces so I didn't have to tie them up, and set off on my run in the same kit I was wearing underneath my wetsuit. It had obviously dried during the ride.

Some people have trouble running after such a long bike ride, but I didn't encounter that problem. We ran through town to get onto the run course. There were a lot of people on the side of the course, which was again very encouraging with everyone shouting. At this point I had my race number on with my name at the bottom, so everyone was shouting, "Come on, Kris!" Pretty cool that people notice that, and they encourage you by your name. Obviously I wanted to put on a decent performance. But I didn't get ahead of myself and try to go at a crazy pace. I looked at my watch and ran the pace that I'm used to—my legs felt good. When I was out there, some people would make comments like, "Those calves are like rockets, man," or, "Those guns should be illegal." But they were positive and encouraging. A couple people would say, "You don't look like an IRONMAN athlete. Good for you." Others recognized me as well. I couldn't believe it—when we were waiting for the swim, some woman came up and she'd been following the video series—she was a personal trainer. There were quite a few people there that I spoke to during the event, before the event, and after the event who recognized me. And it was good that these people who spent a lot of time in the weight room were following the video series, but they'd already started the transition to an IRONMAN anyway.

With the hotter temperatures, I could definitely feel myself getting more thirsty. I had my two 12-ounce bottles on my belt and started going through them pretty quickly—again, with my supplements in there. At every aid station I was getting water, but not only to drink—I was getting it to pour over myself. Whenever they had ice, I grabbed ice and put it down my top in the back and the front just to cool everything down.

It was probably at about mile three that I felt there was definitely a problem in my legs. It was my hip flexors, again. I didn't know if it was just the fatigue setting in, and I wondered, *Is it these bloody tight shorts that are providing resistance every time I pick a leg up?* That's what I blamed it on at the time. I started to become deeply concerned as I approached the aid stations, when all I wanted to do was run but I had no choice but to walk. My legs were absolutely destroyed. Everything else felt good— my asthma didn't play up to the extent that it held me back, my chest and my lungs felt okay. I didn't at any point feel out of breath. I just could not physically pick up my legs. Mentally, I knew I was a strong person, and I was doing everything I could to push my legs to continue jogging. When I did a half-marathon three weeks prior, I was at about a 9-minute pace, but during the Half-IRONMAN I was running about an 11 ½-minute pace. I knew I would still make the cutoff time, but I didn't want to walk it.

I had to get into a mode of just really slowing things down. Walking just before the aid station, all the way through the aid station, and a little bit beyond. I started to drink a lot of water at the aid stations and fill up my bottles because I became so thirsty. Sweat was pouring out of me. It was about 96 degrees. I put on several coats of sunscreen, but I kept sweating it off and still got burnt. Because I was drinking so much, I did have to stop use the porta-loos a few times. I probably lost over 10 minutes there, but I knew I was still within the time limit.

There was such a mental battle going on in that run, and I just couldn't figure out why it was so bad. There were quite a lot of other people walking, but, you know, that didn't comfort me at all. I just felt quite disappointed that I was now shuffling along instead of running. I started talking to myself: *Okay, run to that corner.* When I got to that corner: *Do whatever you can to run to that post.* I'd see someone in the distance with a hosepipe: *Just run to that hosepipe. It will cool you down. You'll get it there. And then when you see the next aid station, that's when you'll walk.*

The self-talk and internal goal-setting kept me going. The run consisted of two laps, so on the second lap I was familiar with milestones to work toward. I knew, *Okay, that's the next point. Okay, I know around this corner is the aid station.* Even though it was so painful in my flexors, nothing else was in pain—my back, my calves—everything was good. My flexors just couldn't pick up my legs.

CROSSING THE FINISH LINE

Even though it was so painful, I was surprised at how fast everything went. During the time, I thought, *Wow, I'm already at mile 8, I'm at mile 10, I've only got three of these miles to go.* It went fast, and I think because there was just so much for the eyes to see. There's so many people out there running with you. There's so many spectators on residential streets—there were gazebos and music; there were microphones; there were hosepipes. People were dressed up. They had signs. It was really awesome to be distracted by all those things—not from the pain so much, but distracted from the mileage that you had to put in and the time you spent out there. Before I knew it, I reached mile 12—and I thought, *What you've got to do is just continue running consistently without stopping now for one more mile.* I was able to do that at a steady pace, and thankfully the main street of Coeur d'Alene is at a decline, so I was able to pick up just a little bit of speed to go over the finish line. With fatigue totally set in, all form and function were destroyed. There was no posture left, no alignment. Luckily, my watch kept me aware of my time and helped me keep pushing.

I crossed the finish line in 6 hours and 19 minutes—two hours ahead of my projected estimation. The time result was surprising and exciting, but I was also concerned because when I finished the last mile, I knew I wouldn't have been able to run another mile farther. My hip flexors were gone. I had nothing left in me. To know I had to double that distance in the full—to spend more time on the bike than the entire race had taken me, *then* run a full marathon—was daunting. In just eight weeks, I would need to perform on an entirely different level.

Up to that point, my training had been perfect to complete a Half-IRONMAN as a larger athlete. It was affirming to learn that my unconventional approach, including the unilateral stability exercises and only 4 hours of cardio training during the work week, had succeeded in keeping me strong, stable, and aligned out on the course. However, I knew that I'd have to step up the game and work on my leg efficiency. A lot more hill repeats, a lot more trail running, more running with ankle weights. I would have to increase my intensity throughout the week, but radically increase volume on the weekends.

When I was in a coffee shop the day after the race, a gentleman came up to me who was an ultramarathon runner. The Half-IRONMAN had been his first triathlon, and he shared that he had struggled significantly on the run as well. This revelation led me to realize that the extreme tightness of my shorts, particularly down my flexors and quads, weren't the only problem; it was exhaustion, plain and simple. I needed to get used to that level of exhaustion through the three disciplines and incorporate more brick sessions of swimming, biking, and running in the same workout. I knew I would be traveling a lot for work in the following weeks, so I needed to get creative to fit all of the necessary training into my schedule. Finishing the half left me with mixed emotions—elation and concern—moving forward.

RACE PREPARATION TIPS

- See an impromptu race that looks like fun? Swap it out for your weekend run and see how all that training is paying off.

- The transitions matter. Keep practicing them so you'll be able to nail them when you're running on fumes come race day.

- Are you training for a race in the heat? Then there's no avoiding it: You must do at least some of your training in the heat. Embrace it—safely. If you live in a colder climate, seek out hot yoga classes and a sauna.

- Make sure you've practiced your nutritional and supplementation approaches extensively. Your stomach won't like surprises on race day!

- Every time you meet someone who has done what you want to do—a seasoned triathlete, for example—learn what you can from them. After all, making speedy transitions from swim to bike during a triathlon is an art unto itself.

CHAPTER 11
TAPERING AND DE-LOADING

As race day approached for the full-length IRONMAN, I felt confident that I'd made the necessary adjustments and my body was ready for the challenge. Two important aspects of training surrounding your event are tapering beforehand and de-loading afterwards.

TAPERING

The tapering process generally begins around three weeks out for most athletes preparing for an endurance event, but for my IRON-MAN I didn't do that. I don't feel that I'm a highly tuned enough triathlete to taper. An endurance athlete of a higher caliber pushes a higher lactate threshold, so it's going to take a longer time to remove the lactic acid and inflammation properly for them. Hybrid athletes following this training program will likely not reach that lactate threshold, so you may not need to taper quite as early as three weeks prior.

My last big ride, swim, and run was two weeks out from the race, which was to prepare me mentally because I hadn't done a 2.4-mile swim matched with a cycle or run up to that point. After I finished that weekend, I began my cardio taper. I slowly brought down my bike and run volume, while maintaining the same volume of swimming. Swimming is nonimpact and doesn't put your body under too much strain. I pulled back the power and speed, but during the last week I swam every day. I didn't do more than 20 miles 3 times per week for the last two weeks, and for my runs they went as high as 6 miles for 3 times per week. I didn't take any days off and filled the rest days with a swim. I brought my calories down ever so slightly because my output was lowered, but I didn't adjust my calories all that much. I was still weight training every day, just not as hard as I usually would, starting a week out. I felt comfortable with this short period of time because I've been weight training for so many years. If you haven't been weight training for over three years, you may want to cut back sooner. I was just trying the finish the IRONMAN as opposed to racing to my peak potential. Listen to your body and listen to your instincts during the taper.

DE-LOADING

My de-load is a little bit different than a lot of other people, because I can't do nothing. I go insane if I can't go out and do something physically exerting. You go from a crazy schedule, composed of getting up early and pushing the three disciplines while continuing weight training as a bodybuilder. That requires a lot of scheduling, discipline, and recovery. If you go from that to nothing, you can easily fall into the abyss. And not only that—you can also get injured. Once Olympic rowers retire, many of them de-load for a minimum of a three-month period to prevent their bodies from seizing up. You shouldn't transition to doing nothing straight after an IRONMAN. It's very important that, before you even finish an event such as an IRONMAN or a marathon, you have another goal immediately planned to follow that event. It will allow you to taper without going too hard or too easy. Personally, I decided to prepare for an ultramarathon to prepare for my de-load.

After the IRONMAN, I took one day off, then I was back in the gym. That was simply to get my body moving again because postrace, the body feels like it's entering rigor mortis—you'll be incredibly sore straight after an event like that. It's very stressful on your body. When you're that stiff, it's easy for your muscles and joints to become dry and brittle. It's important to get the blood flowing into your muscle tissue, tendons, and ligaments. That will improve elasticity and dissipate the scar tissue making you so sore. It will carry nutrients to those areas, which will further speed up the recovery process. Even if you want to sit down and do nothing, you should actually move because that will speed up the recovery process by far. Doing some form of activity—not necessarily weight-bearing activities (if they are weight-bearing, don't train to absolute failure. Train to a maximum of 60 percent failure.)—with high repetitions. Maybe trade off between upper and lower body circuits. We're not trying to evolve and grow at this point; we're trying to detoxify the body and get rid of all the toxins and scar tissue and replenish ourselves. I suggest also doing a form of cardio for at least 30 minutes on a daily basis following an IRONMAN or similar event. Go for an hour or an hour and a half, then bring the time down week by week in ten-minute intervals.

When it comes to de-loading and nutrition, you want to keep your caloric intake quite high for the two days following the IRON-MAN, just to assist with the recovery process because you will go through so many calories on race day. Continue to consume the food and nutrients and fluid in order to bring back up the weight you've lost, then slowly decrease the calories by about 150-200 throughout that week until you come down to your basal metabolic calorie consumption.

I have witnessed thousands of people transform their physiques over a short time period as part of a New Years Resolution, a wedding, a holiday, a bodybuilding competition and photo-shoots, only to put on all the fat they shredded over a 12-plus week timeline in as little as two weeks. When individuals focus on their short-term goals and not the long term, they tend to focus on the destination. Once that destination is met, they stop and all havoc breaks loose. They eat bad, then feel bad, and then eat more in an attempt to release serotonin and endorphins (our "feel-good" hormones) which makes them feel even worse. I am sure you can see the unravelling cycle here.

My suggestion is this: Whatever goal you want to attain following this program, match your calories to your output but do it gradually over a 4-week period. For example, if you want to stop training altogether because you want to take a mental and physical break, decrease your exercise output by 25% and your calories from carbs and fats by 15%. So, your 4-week de-load would look like this:

- Week 1: Decrease cardio by 25% while decreasing calorie consumption from your carbs and fats by 15%

- Week 2: Further decrease cardio by 25% while decreasing calorie consumption from your carbs and fats by 15%

- Week 3: Further decrease cardio by 25% while decreasing calorie consumption from your carbs and fats by 15%

- Week 4: Further decrease cardio by 25% while decreasing calorie consumption from your carbs and fats by 15%

Make sense? The excess in energy that we have mainly used to fuel the MAN of IRON program comes from carbs and fats, so it makes sense that we decrease those two macronutrients. Protein is used for muscle maintenance, collagen production, skin, hair regrowth, eye repair, satiety, and cellular repair amongst many other attributes, so it makes sense to keep protein consumption at around the same levels.

Hydration is also huge part of the recovery, though many people overlook this aspect. Proper hydration transports nutrients around your body to where they're needed. Since your body is made up of about 70 percent fluid, you definitely need to make sure your body is saturated at this time. I don't mean hydrating through solely fluid volume, I mean through electrolytes as well. During this period, you'd want to be taking Hydra-Charge for the electrolytes and anti-oxidants. You'll be experiencing a lot of free radical damage during the event. You'll also want to take fermented glutamine because it helps repair the damaged muscle tissue and helps maintain your immune system. Your immune system will be under a lot of stress and it's very common for people to get sick after a large event like an IRONMAN.

As far as other treatments go, I wouldn't suggest massage right after the race. You'll have a lot of inflammation—in your muscles, your joints, and your connective tissue. Take daily ice baths for about 7-10 days after your IRONMAN. Maybe after your weights workout or cardio, follow up with an ice bath to help rid your body of that inflammation. You won't be able to work toward your next goal until you've recovered. By following a de-load pattern, you're always going to have a much easier time maintaining good fitness, health, mental happiness, longevity, appearance, and long-term goals. The physical process does coincide with the mental process. It's impossible to train at optimal output all year round. Your body needs to periodically take a step back and recover. Mentally, you won't be able to stay motivated all year round, so you need to pull back there too and realign yourself. Regain your composure, come up with another plan of attack for your next event, whatever that may be, and then take the process from there.

"

**IT'S IMPOSSIBLE
TO TRAIN AT OPTIMAL
OUTPUT ALL YEAR
ROUND. YOUR BODY
NEEDS TO PERIODICALLY
TAKE A STEP BACK
AND RECOVER.**

"

TAPERING AND DE-LOADING TIPS

- Race week is the ultimate taper. Rule 1: Don't push it. Rule 2: If you have any doubt about your ability to follow Rule 1, don't lift at all. Just practice what you'll need to have mastered on race day, and make sure your equipment is up to par.

- De-loading is all about limiting inflammation, which is why an ice bath is a perfect inclusion.

- During a de-load, stick to 10-12 reps per set on most moves, even if it means you don't hit failure.

- A proper de-load is all about resisting urges. I'm not great at that—when it comes to not training, at least. Do your best!

CHAPTER 12
RACE DAY, THE FINAL TEST

The thousands of miles completed on the open roads and on my watt bike, the hundreds more put in running along the trails in the Idaho mountains, across cities and countries I had visited over the past 6 months, and the hundreds of thousands of meters swam in open water and in many pools, had come down to this. I was ready. I was calm. From my years of competitive motocross and body-building, I knew my race had been won when nobody was looking during early mornings, late nights, weekends, and times when I didn't want to train. Race day had arrived.

THE PREPARATION

When I went up to Coeur d'Alene, I booked a place 6 miles out of the city to distance myself from the setting of the race and the people. At that point, I was very confident in my ability to finish the race—I just needed to slow everything down to prepare mentally. The brain is a very powerful thing; if the mind is prepared, the body will follow. I listened to slower music, I drove slowly, I breathed slowly, just to calm my nervous system and stay extremely relaxed. I wanted to bring my stress hormones as low as possible. I used the opportunity to do a lot of visualization. When I was body-building professionally, I utilized visualization frequently. I would visualize my impending workout, the clothes I would wear, I'd feel the temperature of the gym, what my muscles would feel like under a certain amount of strain. When I actually went to the gym, I didn't have to motivate myself because I'd already put in the mental work. I wasn't overwhelmed by the prospect of a heavy lift because I knew exactly what to expect.

Up in Coeur d'Alene, I worked to expect the unexpected. I visualized my goggles getting kicked off, my nose being smashed by someone's foot, my tire getting punctured, falling off the bike, my knees hurting on the run, cramping...everything that could go wrong. When it's time to perform, the element of surprise can knock you on your ass. If you're not prepared, you're prepared to fail. I visualized these scenarios so that should they happen, I knew how to deal with them.

The race day was completely fine and nothing happened other than my goggles getting kicked off, but I managed to catch them and put them back on. In the morning, I arrived at the course very early. As I mentioned before, the only time I get nervous is when I don't feel prepared and everything isn't set up. To prevent any race anxiety, I woke up at about 3 a.m., filled up all of my bottles, and made sure my supplements were in order. I prepared all of my food—at least 500 calories per hour to last me through the day. I carried a lot of weight—not only myself, but also all my food and hydration. My pockets were full and I had two bags on the bike. I wanted to make sure I would be recovering during the race and not losing any muscle.

One difference between the half and full IRONMANs is the special needs bags they provide for you to use at mile 77 of the bike and mile 16 of the run. I filled mine with extra fuel and drinks, and a couple of Snickers if I happened to be craving something weird when I reached them. It was nice to have the bags because

IF YOU'RE NOT PREPARED, YOU'RE PREPARED TO FAIL.

I was drinking between 24-32 ounces of water per hour with my supplements.

THE SWIM

When I began training for this event, I felt uneasy in the water, more so in open water, and even more so trapped in a tight wetsuit—now, during the race itself, I was under the stress and nervousness of a race with thousands of others kicking, punching, and jostling for position. Occasionally I felt anxious, but I kept reminding myself of my parents watching and the effort I had put into this. I purposely exhaled underwater, relaxing my mouth and flapping my lips while making a sighing noise. This would help me reset every time I got hit, was blinded by the sun, thought of the distance I yet had to cover, or was attacked by thoughts of quitting and complacency. On my wrist I was able to see the Kara bracelet that was given to me by my good friend Jag Chima at the Golden Temple in Amritsar, India. The temple is full of positive and tranquil vibes, so when I saw it on my wrist during the swim I remembered to stay calm and hydrodynamic, and it reminded me of the Unique Home for Girls Orphanage. The memory gave me another piece of backbone and purpose to make sure I finished what I had embarked on, along with the fact that my parents had come over from Wales to watch the race. Even though it was relaxing and encouraging to have my parents there, it also was more motivating because I didn't want to let them down. When I got out of the water the first time—you get out and run around a cone, then go back in for your second lap—I consumed the energy gel I'd stashed in my cap to knock back 100 calories. During the swim I made sure I stayed to the right of the buoys to stay in a straight line as much as possible. I still was having major problems with my left shoulder, which made it difficult to swim straight, but overall I felt good.

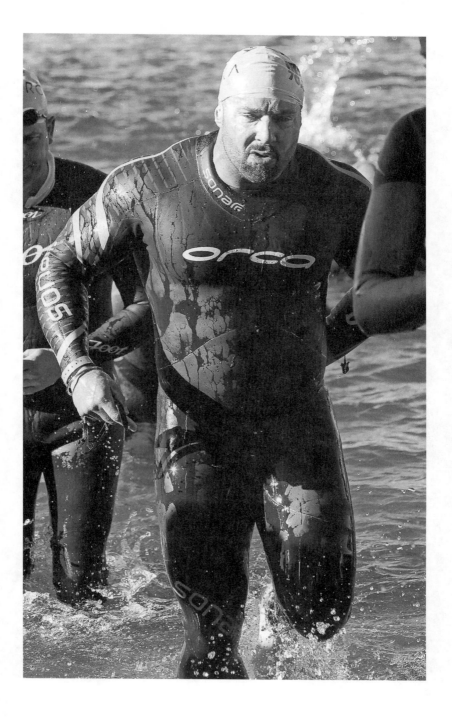

THE BIKE

I took the swim-bike transition very easy and made sure to drink 22 ounces of water with Hydra-Charge so I would be able to store more on my bike. When I started the bike ride there was a competitor next to me cursing because he couldn't clip in. He had accidentally attached his pedals backwards, obviously fitting them back on after dismantling his bike for traveling. I felt bad for him for a split second, because I had my own demons to deal with. I could see that I outweighed a lot of the lean-looking triathletes by around 50-60lbs, and knew we were about to embark on an extremely hilly course.

The bike experience was identical to the Half-IRONMAN for me. I even recognized some of the same competitors who would pass me on the hills and who I would subsequently pass on the flats and downhills. I was surprised to see some overweight people on the bike and thought to myself, *How are these people ahead of me?* I was a little frustrated that people with a bad body composition were ahead, but it quickly dawned on me that they were more buoyant in the water and were much better swimmers than me—they were dropping on the bike ride and all I could see had dropped off by the run.

This time, I made a conscious effort to take it much slower than I did during the Half-IRONMAN. I constantly checked my watch, and had my times from the Half-IRONMAN on my hand to make sure I was pacing slower. All I cared about was finishing. No one would remember if I finished in 12 hours or 16 hours, but they would remember if I didn't cross the finish line. On the bike I focused on pulling with my hamstrings and using my glutes to my advantage rather than just burning out my quads, because I knew I would need the quads a lot on the run. I made a conscious effort to relax my grip and my upper body so I wouldn't use more energy than I needed to. I probably consumed too many calories, truthfully, but I wanted to err on the side of too many than too few. Around five

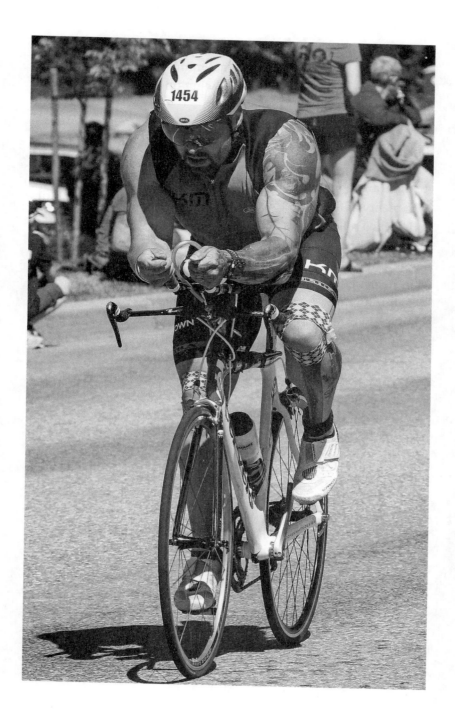

miles before the end of the bike I started increasing the cadence of my pedal stroke so I could somewhat mimic my run. I didn't know what my legs would feel like after being on the bike for 112 miles and a 2.4 mile swim before that.

THE RUN

At the transition I put on my running kit, including a Camelbak with plenty of fluid and food. My legs didn't feel that bad, actually, and it was a relief to start running. I focused on technique: the fore-foot strike, keeping my head up and posture back, maintaining the pendulum swing and a fast cadence. In the Half-IRONMAN I had been surprised by how fast I started running after dismounting the bike, but I figured it was because I was so used to going faster on the bike that the correct running pace simply felt too slow. Determined to prevent myself from making the same mistake, I quickly entered a good rhythm but kept checking my Garmin 920XT watch to stay on pace. I didn't want to walk this time, so I stopped at every single aid station to put ice under my hat, down my top, and down my shorts. As a bigger person, I generate much more heat than the average person, so I wanted to stay cool—it's important for hybrid athletes to keep this in mind. Walking into every aid station, I almost laughed because it felt so good, but to begin running again from each I felt like crying as my hip flexors began to feel the strain.

By the time I reached the midway point of the run, I knew I would finish it, which was a great confidence boost. I had RockTape supporting my tired knees, but they still started to get a bit painful toward the end and my feet developed blisters. Nothing that was going to stop me.

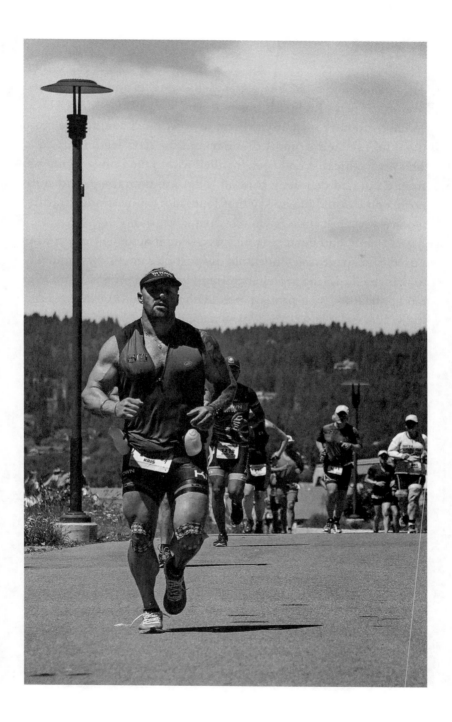

THE FINISH

As I finished across the line, a great sense of relief and pride washed over me as Mike Reilly announced, "you are an IRONMAN." I was so happy to have my parents there to greet me. I couldn't be more thankful for their support that day and the days leading up to it. The work ethic that had been instilled within me from a young age from them had definitely paid off. They are both tough and stubborn, and I would like to say that I am, too. It was strange starting when it was dark, then finishing when it was dark.

My body had been moving for so long it actually hurt to stop. I tried to keep moving while I did my post race interviews. I quickly took in my Re-Kaged protein drink and looked to my girlfriend who fed me healthy, high-protein food. Although the IRONMAN is an individual event, it was certainly a team effort.

LESSONS LEARNED

Overall, I was just happy to finish the race. It's very hard for me to get excited. When I finished, I was actually slightly worried because throughout my entire competitive career—from motocross, to downhill mountain biking, to bodybuilding—race day was always my worst ever day. It didn't matter if I won, because it was still a transition from everything to nothing. It can be very easy for me to fall into the abyss because I no longer had the concrete, tangible purpose and direction to point all of my energy toward. It's so important to have another goal to work toward. One of my favorite things about physical challenges is that each one is a stepping stone to the next. Life is all about experience and adventure. When my life eventually flashes before me, I don't want it to last five minutes. I want it to go on for many, many days. Fit your time with adventure and challenge. It's a gut check; you get to see what

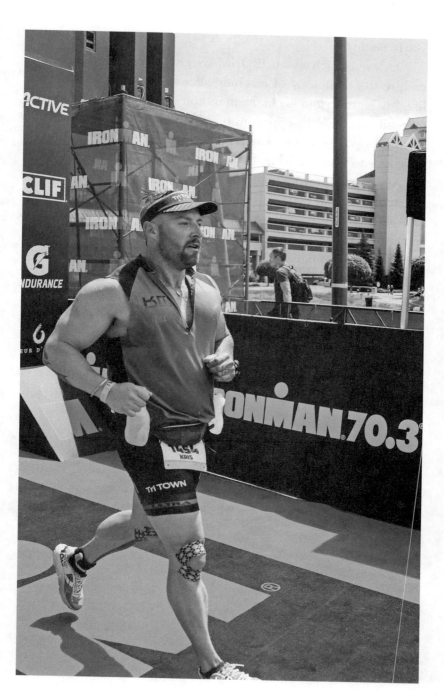

you're made of.

An event such as an IRONMAN gives you the backbone to endure the monotony of reaching success in other parts of your life. You learn to find joy in the monotony, and it's easier to become grateful. You have the opportunity to be bored swimming back and forth in a pool—many people don't have that ability. When you have time to yourself, it creates more space for gratitude.

As I learned throughout out this journey—and hopefully you did, too—you can live as a bodybuilder and as an endurance athlete without losing muscle, possibly even building muscle. But remember, you must supplement and train like a bodybuilder, and especially eat like one. Every endurance athlete should be performing some sort of strength training. Every bodybuilder should be performing some sort of cardio/endurance training. Technique, recovery, and a strong mentality are key.

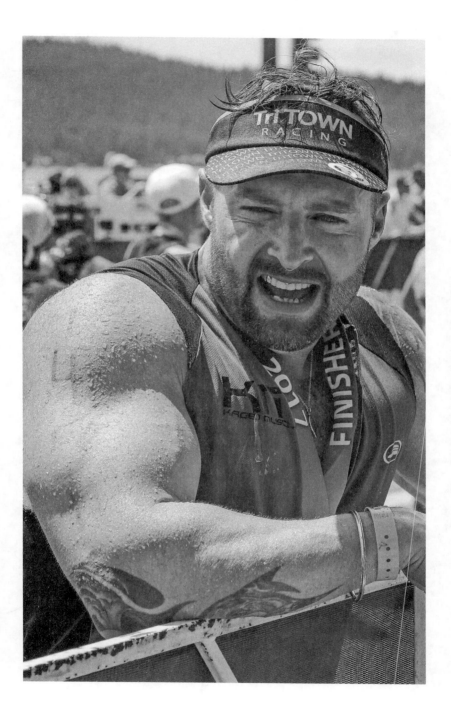

CONCLUSION

In the months after completing the IRONMAN, I have been amazed at the sheer volume of people coming up to me at events and showing me their IRONMAN medals, emailing me, tagging me in photos, and so forth. You can't fake your way through an IRON-MAN—it is incredibly fulfilling and inspiring to interact with so many people who have truly put in the work to accomplish their goal. I am humbled to learn that they joined me on my mission to become a MAN of IRON, and that my journey continues to motivate others even though my race has finished.

Doing this IRONMAN led me to being much more grateful and present in my life. If you're out cycling and running, you have nothing but your thoughts, which is very hard in this day and age when we're used to moving toward our next deadline, our next conference call, our next event scheduled. I've found, and maybe you have too, that this training program leads to the ability to focus more intensely and for longer periods of time. Physical activity releases endorphins, which helps your thoughts head in the positive direction. The combination of focus, holistic health, and positive thinking has changed my life for the better.

Am I hooked to this new Hybrid Athlete way of life? You're damn right I am.

The IRONMAN has changed, expanded, and enlightened my life. I have gained a new group of friends, another form of therapy, a newfound respect for endurance sports, and a great way to actively meditate. Beyond what I've written in this book, all I can do is encourage you to try the same challenge for yourself. What's the downside? You can become healthier, happier, stronger, fitter, more versatile, and inspiring! I guess what I am trying to say is, there is no downside. See you at the finish line where Mike Reilly announces; "_____, you are an IRONMAN."

ABOUT THE AUTHOR

Kris Gethin is a world-renowned body-builder, IRONMAN finisher, ultra-marathoner, CEO of KAGED MUSCLE Supplements, co-founder of the Kris Gethin Gyms franchise, and celebrity personal trainer. He travels the globe hosting fitness seminars, workshops, exhibitions, and training the best of the best. Passing on his knowledge and techniques to his fans and followers, Kris has transformed millions of physiques through his video series you can find online.

He is the author of numerous bestselling books, including *Body by Design, The Adventures of KAGED MUSCLE,* and *The Transformer.* Kris is also the founder of the DTP training method, former editor-in-chief for Bodybuilding.com, and director of trainers for Physique Global. As the CEO of KAGED MUSCLE, Kris has elevated the brand to be the highest-rated and reviewed supplement company in the world. Kris is originally from Wales in the United Kingdom but currently resides in Boise, Idaho.

ACKNOWLEDGMENTS

My girlfriend, Sunshine. Your smiles, laughs, and company during our training and adventures are memories I'll never forget. Thank you for joining me for two of the 70.3 IRONMANs and being a major part in my life. You are my Iron-Woman.

My nieces, Alys and Magi. You give me so much joy watching your unprecedented innocence, honesty, and humor. I feel that I learn from you instead of you learning from me.

Mum and Dad, thanks for enduring yet another physical challenge taken upon by myself. Traveling from Wales to the U.S. to support me during my IRONMAN meant more to me than you'll ever know.

To all the little souls from the All Girls Orphanage in India who I did this for, you gave me the accountability to persevere when I had doubt. The Kara on my wrist reminded me several times during the IRONMAN that you are all so much bigger than I am.

My coaches, Alex Viada and Mike Fecik. Your expertise, guidance, and instinctive adaptation took me from a very un-fit asthmatic bodybuilder to Hybrid Athlete and IRONMAN finisher in six months. You've now introduced me to a different world of possibilities.

Antonio and the entire TriTown crew. The guidance, bike set-up, mechanical abilities, support on the course, introduction to the local triathlon community, and friendship I've gained from you all is priceless. I can't say the same for the lactate threshold tests you put me though.

My formulator, Brian Rand at KAGED MUSCLE supplements. Your scientific, strategic creation of my supplant stacks during these six months were incredible. Bodybuilding with crazy intensity five days per week whilst training for an IRONMAN, and adding several pounds of muscle in the process, wouldn't have been possible without your unbelievable talent to help me recover and perform.

My close friend and business partner, Jag Chima, thank you for making this book partnership happen. Your loyalty and selflessness is unbelievable and I keep learning from you daily. One thing I did learn is not to do a 1,000 mile bike ride across India within the space of a week. I don't think you'll ever recover.

My close friend, Ray Klerk, for your support and guidance during the editorial process. You helped take this book to the next level and I'm truly grateful for that.

My cousin, Adam Gethin, for your unparalleled determination to put this book into the hands of every person that needs it. We couldn't have reached the masses without your marketing prowess and ingenuity.

Last and not least, my unbelievable ghost writer Rachel and publisher Bobby. Rachel, your patience, commitment, work ethic, and talent to translate my gibbering attempt at the English language to what I see in this book is honorable to witness! I am so grateful for you. Your decision to support this book, Bobby, especially following the first "unpredicted collapse," is something I'll always remember. Your belief to bring my idea to reality is appreciated by myself and thousands of others who will read these pages.

RESOURCES

If you're interested in learning more about my process and the research materials I used in my MAN of IRON journey, I have included this list of resources for your reference.

- www.krisgethin.com
- www.kagedmucle.com
- RunTri.com
- *The Training Bible* by Joe Friel
- *Iron War* by Matt Fitzgerald
- *How Bad Do You Want It?* by Matt Fitzgerald
- *The Well-Built Triathlete* by Matt Dixon
- *A Life Without Limits* by Chrissie Wellington
- *To the Finish Line* by Chrissie Wellington
- *The Grace to Race* by Sister Madonna Buder
- *The Unlikely Finisher 140.6* by Dale Petelinsek
- *Iron Cowboy* by James Lawrence
- *You are an IRONMAN* by Jaques Steinberg
- *The Time Crunched Triathlete* by Carmichael and Rutberg
- *100 Bedtime Stories for Triathletes* by Allan Pitman
- *As the Crow Flies* by Craig Alexander
- *17 Hours of Glory* by Mathias Muller and Timothy Carlson
- *Redemption* by John McAvoy
- *Operation IRONMAN* by George Mahood
- *Swim Bike Run* by the Brownlee Brothers
- *Relentless Forward Progress* by Bryon Powell
- *Born to Run* by Christopher Dougall

NOTES

1. Proposition 65 Office of Environmental Health Hazard Assessment, State of California. Retrieved from https://oehha.ca.gov/proposition-65 2016

2. Støren, O., Helgerud, J., Støa, E. M., Hoff, J. (June 2008). *Medicine and Science in Sports and Exercise.* Trondheim, Norway. 40(6):1087-92. Retrieved from https://www.ncbi.nlm.nih.gov/pubmed/18460997

3. Park B. J., Tsunetsugu, Y., Kasetani, T., Kagawa, T., Miyazaki, Y. (Jan 2010). *Environmental Health and Preventative Medicine.* Center for Environment, Health and Field Sciences, Kashiwa, Chiba, Japan. 15(1):18-26. Retrieved from https://www.ncbi.nlm.nih.gov/pubmed/19568835

4. Participation trends in ultra-endurance sports (2017). Ultra Sports Science. 30 May, 2017. Denver, CO.

5. Andersen, C. A., Clarsen, B., Johansen, T. V., Engebretsen, L. (Sept 2013). *British Journal of Sports Medicine.* 47(13):857-61. Retrieved from https://www.ncbi.nlm.nih.gov/pubmed/23902775 Oslo Sports Trauma Research Center, Norwegian School of Sport Sciences, Norway.

6. Folland, J. P., Allen, S. J., Black, M. I., Handsaker, J.C., & Forrester, S. E. (July 2017). *Medicine and Science in Sports and Exercise.* Loughborough, United Kingdom. 49(7):1412-1423. Retrieved from https://www.ncbi.nlm.nih.gov/pubmed/28263283

7. Pattinson, C. L., Allan, A. C., Staton, S. L., Thorpe, K. J., & Smith, S. S. (2016). Environmental Light Exposure Is Associated with Increased Body Mass in Children. PLoS ONE 11(1): e0143578. Retrieved from https://doi.org/10.1371/journal.pone.0143578

ADDITIONAL TITLES
BY KRIS GETHIN

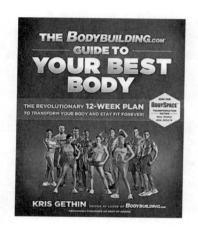

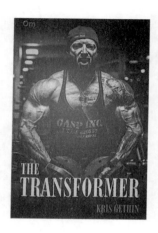

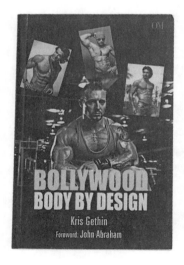